Back Pain: It's All in Your Neck

David B. Tuchinsky, D.C.

Writers Club Press
New York Lincoln Shanghai

Back Pain: It's All in Your Neck

Writers Club Press
an imprint of iUniverse, Inc.

iUniverse books may be ordered through booksellers or by contacting:

iUniverse
2021 Pine Lake Road, Suite 100
Lincoln, NE 68512
www.iuniverse.com
1-800-Authors (1-800-288-4677)

ISBN-13: 978-0-595-00623-6
ISBN-10: 0-595-00623-X

Printed in the United States of America

Dedicated to my loving parents, Nathan and Judith Tuchinsky and my father-in-law Albert Levite.

Contents

Chapter 1

Introduction: Health is Balance

Overview

Do your heels wear out unevenly? This may indicate an uneven leg length, which will cause stress along the spine.

Do you "crack" your neck, back or other joints frequently? If so, your spinal column may be out of alignment, forcing other joints to compensate and pop frequently.

Do your feet flare when walking? If your feet are not parallel (both facing forward) there may be a problem with the lower spine or hips.

Do you feel stiffness in the back or neck? Subluxations may cause stress to muscles by forcing them to tense frequently.

Do you have bad posture? If you stand on two bathroom scales, you can see if you carry your weight in an unbalanced way, forcing the spine to curve to one side or the other. Slouching, too, can cause vertebral damage over time or force a disk to bulge backward.

This list, while cursory, gives us a gleaning into how chiropractors assess the health of the spine.

The importance of the spine is embedded in our very language. We speak of the weak as "spineless" and the strong as having "backbone." A good horror movie is "spine-tingling." Even this book is held together with a "spine."

However, these are merely dead metaphors. They have, through end-less repetition, lost their freshness, and we cease to see them as metaphors. In the same way, the spine itself has become invisible. Its seamless functioning rarely crosses our minds and if so, only when it falters. Back pain, while it alerts us to the importance of the spine, is quickly forgotten when the pain vanishes. Yet back pain has reached nearly epidemic levels in the United States. Eight out of every ten Americans suffer at least one episode of debilitating back pain in their lifetimes. Over one million workdays are lost to back pain at a cost of over $50 billion annually. It is for this reason that chiropractic is a vital form of health care.

The reason for the wave of back pain lies in the nature of habit. It is easy to ignore the spine because it is synonymous with both strength and flexibility. We form habits that, over time, inflict damage on our backs. We realize it only too late, when we are immobilized or hunched in pain. We can, however, be aware of our habits, and alter them accordingly. In this sense, chiropractic is more than just treatment. It is a system that uses the body's own healing ability to restore and *maintain* good health.

In the following chapters, our goal is to explore the main procedures of treating and preventing back pain. We hope to provide a basic guide to the causes, treatment, and prevention of back pain. In order to present useful information, we will give only glancing attention to chiropractic's history and status. We encourage the reader to investigate these sociological issues independently. This text, while it recognizes the importance of these concerns, focuses on making the reader more aware of chiropractic's benefits by exploring the roots and solutions of back pain itself.

The State of Chiropractic

Although there is still friction between mainstream medicine and chiropractic, there is also growing acceptance. In the last twenty years, the number of chiropractors in the U.S. has increased by 48 percent, resulting in more than 58,000 in practice today. Some surveys estimate that around 40 million Americans visited a chiropractor in 1997.

Why such a dramatic increase? Part of the answer lies in the willingness of insurance companies to pay for chiropractic treatments. In the last few decades, too, favorable legislation has paved the way. In all, there is new acceptance of chiropractic, although this was not always so. Since its founding in1895 by Daniel David Palmer, chiropractic has sustained fierce criticism. Chiropractors were seen as charlatans and hacks.

Today however, despite lingering dissent, chiropractic has found credibility. In all 50 states, chiropractors must be licensed and must hold degrees from accredited chiropractic schools. They must receive at least six years of education and training to be licensed. Many obtain further degrees in specialized fields such as radiology, sports medicine, or neurology. Overall, more and more mainstream doctors see chiropractic as a legitimate health care system.

What is Chiropractic?

Chiropractic, quickly defined, involves the precise manipulation of the spinal column to allow the body to heal itself more quickly. How does the spine relate to overall health? To understand this, we must first explore one of the central notions of chiropractic: that is, the body has built-in recuperative abilities. Chiropractors often use the term *innate intelligence* to describe the body's inborn ability to heal itself. When this natural mechanism is working, cells are replaced, tissues re-grown, and infections quelled. This concept, central to chiropractic, means that the body tends toward a state of equilibrium, or *homeostasis*. If there is an imbalance—an infection or injury—the body seeks to rectify it.

How does the spine relate to homeostasis? The spinal cord, as the coordinator of the nervous system, affects every part of the body. When there is a disturbance in the spine, the parts of the body under its control can suffer. One famous illustration of this can be seen in the story of a patient treated by chiropractic's founder, D.D. Palmer in 1895. He wrote that the patient had been deaf for 17 years that he could not hear the racket of a wagon on the street or the ticking of a watch. I...was informed that when he was exerting himself in a cramped, stooping position, he felt something give way in his back and immediately became deaf. An examination showed a vertebra racked from its normal position. I racked it into position by using spinous process as a lever and soon the man could hear as before.

This extraordinary case led D.D. Palmer to develop a specific technique for adjustment. But the true significance of the story is that it illustrates chiropractic's central aim: by carefully adjusting the spine, the nervous system is given a better opportunity to restore health in the rest of the body.

Evidence of how heavily the body relies on the nervous system can be found in the case of the Windsor autopsies. In the early 1920s, a medical doctor named Henry Windsor questioned the principles of chiropractic. He therefore demanded evidence that the rest of the body's functions can be affected by a defective spinal column. He dissected the cadavers of 75 humans and 72 cats. In each case, he looked for a correlation between variations in the spinal column and disease elsewhere in the body. His results, published in "The Medical Times," showed that in all cases, a particular disease could be traced to the part of the spine that controls that organ. For instance, he found that for all 20 cases of heart disease, malfunctions existed in the section of spine that controls the heart. In examining diseases of the liver, stomach, and lungs, he found the same 100 percent correlation between the disease and the corresponding spinal section.

While the Windsor autopsies are not the final word on chiropractic, they indicate that the underlying principles of chiropractic are finding increasing validation. The findings also indicate that further investigation is needed. Indeed, studies that have been done since Windsor have fortified his findings.

With this in mind, we continue our definition of chiropractic as a method of assisting the body's natural tendency to heal. When, through misuse or accident, the spine becomes unbalanced, the chiropractor becomes an essential agent in steering the process of self-healing. Discomfort is the body's way of flagging deeper problems. Neck strain, headaches, and lower back pain are signals that something is awry in the spine. By addressing the possible causes of these effects in the spinal column, the chiropractor intercepts the problem and prevents it from showing up as pain.

This approach distinguishes chiropractic from mainstream medicine. M.D.s often seek to alleviate the symptoms without addressing their cause. They will prescribe a drug, say aspirin for a headache, and if the pain goes away, the problem is dismissed. This is *not* to say that M.D.s are reckless. Indeed, the aim of both medical and chiropractic doctors is the same: to heal. Further, there are many times when medical doctors *do* treat the root of an ailment. There is, however, a fundamental difference in approach. In general, mainstream medicine views the body as a machine, composed of complex, but distinct parts that can break down. The medical doctor becomes, in this sense, a mechanic. Chiropractors, however, see the body as a self-healing whole that is coordinated through the nervous system. They offer a method of allowing this system to correct itself, without invasive techniques.

These differing points of view give us two rather different methods of health care. M.D.s most often focus on treating the patient with drugs, hoping to fight off an invading infection. The chiropractor, however, attempts to head off the *cause* of the dysfunction by looking for its origin in the spinal column.

Another difference between mainstream medicine and chiropractic is in the way they view a healthy body. Often, M.D.s see a patient as either sick or well. If an infection is absent, then the patient is considered healthy. Chiropractic doctors see a patient's health as appearing along a *continuum*. In this model, a patient is healthy only in the sense that he is at the top of this spectrum of health. Ideal health can degenerate by gradual degrees into eventual chronic ill health. Along this continuum, the flexibility and resilience of the spine is compromised, making damage more likely. The continuum concept is important to chiropractic philosophy of correcting the root of a problem. Because a patient appears somewhere on this scale at all times, the maintenance of the spine is always a concern. The patient, seeing the possibility of sinking into chronic ill health, is more likely to take measures to prevent it. In the medical model, a patient can be fixed, dismissed, and deemed automatically healthy. The problem is then forgotten, thus making it more likely that it will reoccur.

Despite these basic differences, chiropractors and M.D.s often work in conjunction. For this reason, most chiropractors are considered *portal of entry* practitioners. That is, they do not pretend to cure every affliction, and they don't pretend that chiropractic, while a very good method of health care, is the only one. Further, portal of entry status means that if any serious problems are even suspected, the chiropractor will refer the patient to another medical professional. In all, the strength of chiropractic lies in its ability to satisfy the patient in specific areas of health, namely the spine. Chiropractic has seen tremendous success in the healing of lower back pain and whiplash.

Another distinctive quality of chiropractic is that because it is concerned with the patient's whole system, there is a greater tendency to work closely with the patient. Many people find great satisfaction in the process, and tend to heal faster. An M.D. on the other hand, while working under the same intention to heal, may tend to prescribe drugs to mask the pain of a lower back ailment, without correcting the root of the problem. This approach lengthens the healing process, and creates frustration for the patient.

Overall, chiropractic is usually defined in opposition to mainstream medicine. It is a drugless, natural way to heal a patient. It not only corrects problems when they occur, but also promotes the overall health of the spine. This, in turn, encourages health in the rest of the body.

The Specifics

Having seen the main rationale of chiropractic, we can turn to the specific methods of the practice. What do chiropractors do? What can you expect from a chiropractor, and how can you benefit?

Before answering these questions, we must briefly cover some basic anatomy. The terms that follow, while they may seem technical, are easily mastered. Following this, we'll address whacking and cracking, and other misleading terms.

We begin with a portrait of the spinal column. It is a chain of 24 movable bones called *vertebrae*. These vertebrae are separated by flexible shock absorbers called *disks*. This much is familiar to many of us, as is the profile of the spine. From the front or back, a healthy spine is straight. From the side, we can see the familiar spinal shape. Beginning at the base of the skull, the spine curves forward slightly in what is called a *lordosis*. Along the ribs, the spine curves backward, and below the ribs, it curves forward in another lordosis. The top seven vertebrae are called the *cervical* vertebrae. The middle twelve, where the ribs are attached, make up the *thoracic* region. The bottom five make up the *lumbar* region. These lower vertebrae join to a large bone called the *sacrum*. Below this, we find the pointed bone called the *coccyx*.

The curves of the spine form when we are infants. At that age, our backs were shaped like the letter C. As we learned to crawl, the lumbar curve formed, sagging downward. This system, while it worked well for a crawling beast, was soon called upon to support us when we learned to stand. The result of this inevitable step is that the spine, though strong, is vulnerable to misalignment.

The Spine Gone Awry

Despite the resiliency of the spine, problems often arise. When, for example, the natural curves of the spine are pushed beyond their limits, we experience a *hyperlordosis*, a condition characteristic of a slumped posture. People with pot bellies or poor abdominal muscles experience this. In hyperlordosis, the spine is straightened, and the disks between the vertebrae are allowed to bulge backward.

One of the main problems chiropractic addresses is *subluxation,* or the misalignment of vertebrae. D.D. Palmer wrote that subluxation "perpetuates disease." Today, we know that misalignment can cause imbalances in the nervous impulses channeled through the spine. The result of subluxation is often an overabundance of nervous signals. We can see an example of this overproduction when we witness a car crash: with mental stress, we produce more adrenaline than is needed, and we begin to shake, with no outlet for the nervousness. The same imbalance can happen with a subluxation: an overactive nervous system wreaks havoc with the rest of the body. Similarly, though less common, a *suppressed* nervous system can cause problems. In the words of D.D. Palmer: "…too much or not enough energy is disease."

To understand how a subluxation alters the nervous system, we must again briefly cover some anatomy. Vertebrae provide both flexibility and strength, and are perfectly suited for housing the spinal cord. The fin-like bones on each vertebra, or *facet joints,* help guide movement of the spine. The spinal cord runs through the center of each vertebra, with nerve roots emerging from both sides of the vertebrae, between the facet joints.

Facet joints are covered in a thin layer of highly sensitive cartilage. Since this makes them vulnerable, they are a common source of back pain. They are called the "storm center" of the spine for this reason. In a similar, but much less common case, the nerve itself can become irritated by calcium build-up along the edges of the vertebrae, called bone spurs.

An unbalanced spine—one curved beyond its natural shape—is prone to subluxations. When the vertebrae are unaligned, the nearby nerves may become irritated. Often, people use the term "pinched nerve" to describe this problem. The term is inaccurate, however, even if doctors sometimes use it for simplicity. However, the nerves along the spine are rarely pinched, a serious trauma causing only about 10 to 15 percent of spinal problems. Most problems happen when malfunction-ing vertebrae *irritate* the nerve, stimulating the nervous system too much. We have seen the damage this can inflict on the spine, and on the rest of the body. D.D. Palmer was one of the earliest to recognize that since the nerves are given ample room to move within the vertebrae, an actual pinching of the nerve is rare. Of course, simple back pain is the most direct consequence of a "pinched nerve."

In a similar problem, the disks between vertebrae account for much back pain. Here, the term "slipped disk" is applied to back pain, but this is another inaccurate term. The disk can tear, bulge or even rupture. But because the way it is cushioned between the vertebrae, they cannot slip.

To understand problems with the disks, envision the disk as a jelly doughnut. Inside, there is a thick substance called the *nucleus*. This cen-ter is surrounded by an elastic ring of fibers called the *annulus fibrosis*. Problems occur when this layer decays from the inside outward, form-ing weaknesses or even cracks. In the worst cases, the jelly doughnut oozes its contents. The nucleus can escape and displace the nerve root. This can cause pain that extends to the legs and feet. But more likely than a rupture, a disk may bulge and excite nearby nerves. Bulging of disks comes from long-term trauma associated with slouching, bad sleeping habits or repetitive tasks that tax the spine's flexibility. Sometimes, a single accident can harm a disk, but if a disk is unhealthy to begin with, it will be more likely to suffer injury.

Another spinal problem is called *scoliosis*. Looking at a spine from the rear, it should appear straight. Scoliosis is an *unnatural* sideways curve of the spine. It is thought that scoliosis occurs according to a per-son's heredity. It may also be the result of an injury. For the most part, scoliosis appears in children and young adults as an unevenness in the shoulders or lower back pain. If scoliosis goes undetected, it can worsen in a person's twenties, after the spine as reached its full growth. Traditional medicine treats this with braces or surgery. If detected early, however, a chiropractor is able to affect specific spinal adjustments to achieve excellent results.

The Decline of the Spine: Habits and Tips

Having seen how the spine functions, we can turn to habits that harm the spine, and tips on how we can alter those habits for the better. First, however, ask yourself the following questions to get an idea of your spinal health:

1) Do your heels wear out unevenly? This may indicate an unevenleg length, which will cause stress along the spine.

2) Do you "crack" your neck, back or other joints frequently? If so, your spinal column may be out of alignment, forcing other joints to compensate and pop frequently.

3) Do your feet flare when walking? If your feet are not parallel (both facing forward) there may be a problem with the lower spine or hips.

4) Do you feel stiffness in the back or neck? Subluxations may cause stress to muscles by forcing them to tense frequently.

5) Do you have bad posture? If you stand on two bathroom scales, you can see if you carry your weight in an unbalanced way, forcing the spine to curve to one side or the other. Slouching, too, can cause vertebral damage over time or force a disk to bulge backward.

We might add to this list a general feeling of fatigue or uneasiness. Although fatigue can result from many things, it may indicate that the body is using some of its energy to correct an unbalanced spinal column. If the spine is aligned, then the body can direct its energy toward more productive tasks.

How, then, do we throw our spines off balance? The short answer is we do it everyday, without thinking about it. Most spinal injuries are the result not of a single accident, but of habitual misuse. Take sitting, for example, an apparently innocent and harmless activity. When standing, we put about 25 pounds of pressure on our backs. Sitting, however, puts almost 250 pounds of pressure on the spine. Imagine all the time you spend sitting at work, at home or in the car. A good recommendation is to take stretch breaks to restore the natural spinal curves and relieve muscle tension.

Another way we throw our backs off kilter is by twisting and turning our backs in daily life. A repetitive twisting motion, such as reaching for items around your desk, stresses and shears the facet joints on the vertebrae.

The cliché about lifting with your legs is a cliché for a reason: by bending the spine forward to an unnatural degree, there is a risk that the disks will bulge backward, stressing them. One should minimize the reaching distance to objects at work. Any activity that requires repetitive twisting or movement of the head should be arranged to reduce these movements.

Sleeping habits, too, can affect our spines. Because we spend one third of our lives sleeping, we have ample opportunity to inflict spinal damage. In fact, many patients complain of back pain in the morning, having gone to bed feeling fine. Sleeping in a fetal position, for example, reverses the primary curves of the spine, stressing the vertebrae. Lying on your stomach, too, can twist the upper, cervical vertebrae because the head is rotated ninety degrees. The best sleeping posture is lying on your side so that your spine is straight. When lying on your back, your head should be on an even level, not angled forward or backward.

In subsequent chapters, we will explore these and other tips in more detail. In general, use your common sense. A bad posture will clearly have detrimental effects over time. Weak back and stomach muscles make you less able to maintain a healthy posture. The long-term consequences could be pain and loss of mobility. One of the primary aims of chiropractic is to help people form better habits to reduce the possibility of injury, rather than fixing it after it has happened. This is, in the long run, more effective and cheaper.

What to Expect

A popular way to refer to chiropractic is "whacking and cracking." While this may sound menacing, the truth is that most chiropractors are not in the torture business. Most of them work through precise and gentle adjustments that are soundless. There is nothing haphazard or brutal about it. When the infamous popping sound *is* heard, as does happen, it is the sound of air rushing in to fill the gap when a joint is slightly separated.

An insight into the specific techniques of chiropractic is important to anyone considering it. We will cover these in detail later, but we can get an introduction by looking at two different types of chiropractors, namely "mixers" and "straights."

Some chiropractors tend to follow the doctrine of D.D. Palmer very closely. These "straights" represent the minority of chiropractors. They rely solely on adjustments of the spine to boost the body's innate intelligence. These doctors seek to heal the entire body through spinal adjustments, including alleviating headaches or simply helping the patient feel more energetic.

Most chiropractors, however, are "mixers." That is, they combine spinal adjustment with other techniques such as massage, hot packs, or nutritional counseling. They will occasionally recommend herbal or vitamin remedies and some will even do acupuncture. Mixers are more likely than straights to work with a medical doctor, and will limit their practice to bone, nerve, and muscle problems. Many mixers have specialties, such as sports medicine, and hold degrees in that area.

Clearly, the techniques of these two types vary. But both see the crucial role the spine plays in overall health. Even if the chiropractor focuses only on lower back pain, he or she will always be interested in finding the least invasive way to heal. Neither will use drugs or surgery.

The basic chiropractic principle of achieving homeostasis, or a balance within the body, applies to both types.

When visiting a chiropractor, you can expect a careful screening of your medical history. The doctor will examine you for range of motion and other conditions that can harm the spine. If there is any doubt that a condition could be the result of a serious problem, such as a brain tumor, certain degenerative diseases, or anything that would require major surgery, the chiropractor will refer you to a medical doctor.

However, if the ailment is within the realm of chiropractic, the doctor will perform further tests, including a *palpation* test for swelling. This test involves scanning the spinal column by touch to detect abnormalities.

Many chiropractors will use x-rays to both verify their diagnoses and look for possible complications before proceeding with treatment. Most chiropractors have extensive training in taking x-rays.

Having gained as much information as possible, the chiropractor will recommend a treatment program. Treatment times vary, depending on the severity of the affliction. In fact, a study done by the RAND Corporation indicated that a short-lived lower back problem could be eliminated in usually about six weeks. Some more complicated problems have seen treatment times as varied as six to sixteen weeks.

In all, the chiropractic treatment aims at working closely with the patient. Regardless of the techniques used, any chiropractor will stress the doctor-patient relationship. Patients with a positive outlook will be more likely to focus their attention on healing, rather than on frustration or anger.

Summary

Because the spine serves its purpose seamlessly, we often forget that it is vulnerable. Back pain, then, results from habits that ignore the health of the spine. Consequently, there is an epidemic of spinal problems in the U.S. today. Chiropractic seeks to use the body's natural defenses by correcting problems in the spinal column, which is the main coordinator of the body. The art of chiropractic centers on the notion that a balanced spine can promote health without use of drugs or surgery. A balanced spine is a healthy one. Any variation or imbalance in the spine can have consequences, if not in the spine itself, in other parts of the body. The chiropractor becomes an important agent in directing the body's natural defenses. While the advantages of chiropractic can be enormous, they are also very specific. Chiropractic can heal back pain in a very gentle and accurate way.

In the following chapters, we will seek to arm the reader with an understanding of chiropractic that will help to assess its benefits. Only with a careful examination of its procedures can chiropractic be given its full due.

Chapter 2

The Roots of Back Pain

Introduction

Back pain often seems unpredictable. It may happen after lifting a small bag of groceries or after doing strenuous yard work. You may go to bed feeling fine, but awake in pain. This apparently random nature of back pain can leave you feeling helpless, vulnerable, and frustrated. Although the source of this kind of pain is often unknown, we can identify some of the primary suspects. Back pain is a complex thing, and no one source accounts for all of it. However, by examining the most likely sources of spinal trauma—whether by misuse or accident—we can reduce the probability of future damage. Certainly, damage to the spine is often unavoidable. However, it proves more efficient in the long run to *prevent* the damage rather than remedy it later.

In this chapter, we will expand on some of the issues raised in the introduction. We will look closely at the causes of different types of back pain. We will see that a spinal malfunction can yield a variety of problems, such as acute back pain, pain in the legs or hips, and even headaches. The severity of back pain ranges from merely annoying to excruciating. Overall, back pain has become a costly epidemic in the United States. An estimated $50 to $75 billion is spent on back pain annually. Add to this the reduced quality of life for millions of people.

Given these stakes, it is important to illuminate the causes of back pain as a first step toward preventing it.

Types of Pain

While back pain can result from many things, it comes primarily from trauma inflicted on the spine or surrounding muscles. We define trauma here broadly: any stress that causes a malfunction in the operation of the spine. This stress may be the result of a single accident or the accumulation of many small traumas. Consider, for instance, the case of back pain resulting from a car wreck. The acute neck pain, called whiplash, comes from a sudden and violent jarring. This is what most of us ordinarily think of as trauma. However, damage may also seem to have no apparent source. The pain may indicate a repetitive strain injury, most often associated with work-related problems such as carpal tunnel syndrome. In general, back pain can result from habitual misuse or a single incident. Various factors within these two categories can cause back pain:

- Muscle strain or spasms.
- Heredity.
- Aging or degeneration.
- Irritated nerves.
- Pain referred from other areas of the body—or *trigger* point injuries.
- Poor posture.
- An auto accident.
- A bad fall, no matter how long ago.
- Excess weight.
- Inactivity.
- Poor muscle tone, especially in the abdominal area.
- Emotional or chemical stress.

Certainly, problems in the spine ordinarily show up as pain near the faulty spot along the spine. However, other symptoms can point to spinal imbalance as well. Shoulder pain, headaches, eyestrain, or even lack of energy can indicate a spinal malfunction. In addition, a painful condition known as *sciatica* can result from the bulging of a disk between vertebrae. Sciatica is pain that travels along the sciatic nerve, running down the back of the leg from the hip to the foot. This pain is often described as numbness, tingling, or sometimes a burning sensation. It has been described as hot water running down the back of the legs.

Pain is merely the body's way to flag deeper problems. Whether the pain appears in the back, legs, or head, it may often be treated with precise adjustments of the vertebrae. By addressing the root of the pain, not only will a patient be relieved from suffering, but will be less likely to relapse. If the significance of the pain is ignored, the body may suffer further damage in the spine or even other regions. To understand this danger, we must briefly reiterate the central notions of spinal adjustment.

A Glance Back: Approaches to Health Care

Although we have already explored the central notions of chiropractic in relation to mainstream medicine, it is important to apply them to the specific causes of back pain. We explored two rather different approaches to healing. One is the medical or *allopathic* approach. The other is the chiropractic, or the *vertebral adjustment* approach. To understand chiropractic, it must be placed within the context of healing arts in general. It is best defined in contrast to traditional medicine. While many texts engage in debate on this topic, our interest is merely to define the philosophy of each. Only by understanding the larger picture can we begin to examine the specifics of back pain and its treatment.

We turn first, then, to allopathy. This approach seeks to heal the body with methods based on the germ theory of illness. It sees the body as a victim of invading microbes that are to be fended off through various surgical or medicinal methods. While there are certainly many conditions that demand such an approach, the fundamental philosophy often neglects some important issues. For example, there is evidence that microbes—influenza or tuberculosis—may become resistant to immunization over long periods. These microbes have tremendous adaptive powers. That is, the strains killed off by the medicine leave the field clear for a heartier strain, which then reproduces with greater speed. Without competition from the weaker strains, the stronger strains thrive. In this sense, immunization may actually worsen matters in the end. Philosopher Virgil Strang, D.C. (hon.) expresses this notion:

How utterly foolish, wasteful and bankrupt to think that we should build a health care system upon an infinite stream of potions, each of which is destined to be quickly discarded.

In a similar problem, the body often forms a resistance to strong medications taken for headaches. Substances such as caffeine—an ingredient in many medications—have been shown to aggravate headaches if taken for long periods. People with chronic headaches often take strong painkillers to relieve their symptoms. This can lead to a drug dependency that may ultimately serve to worsen their pain.

What we hope to illustrate here is that the allopathic approach tends to mask the pain rather than address its root cause. Granted, mainstream medicine exerts considerable effort to identify the roots of many serious problems, such as cerebral hemorrhages or tumors. Further, all medical doctors would agree that preventing ailments is less costly in the long run than patching them up later. However, there remains in society and medicine an underlying mentality that if the symptom disappears, then the patient is cured. While this may seem adequate, it ignores the possibility that neglected problems could re-emerge as severe pain in the future.

Recall that chiropractic's approach focuses on finding and treating the cause of the pain, which can often be traced to the spine. Because the spinal column is the coordinator of the body, a faulty spine can have adverse consequences for systems far from the spine itself. The most common problem is a subluxation, or a misalignment of vertebrae. This imbalance can wreak havoc with the central nervous system, thus impinging the body's natural ability to heal. The doctor of chiropractic applies precise diagnosis and treatment to the affected vertebra or disk.

The following case report shows a patient who tried both medical and chiropractic approaches:

A nineteen-year-old female had a long history of chronic headaches that grew more severe over four years. Her symptoms included migraine headaches and dizziness. In addition, she experienced chills, sweats, insomnia, a stiff neck, and shoulder pain. When these symptoms first began four years previously, the patient visited both a gynecologist and general practitioner. Various medications were given to relieve the pain, including Fiorinal, Codeine, and an oral contraceptive. While she found some short-lived relief, she reported that they didn't seem to help much. She described the pain as stiff and tight. The headaches occurred so frequently—as many as five a week—that they blended into one continuous episode.

After receiving a massage from a friend that eased her pain, the patient went to a chiropractor. An examination of the spine revealed tenderness in the upper five vertebrae. There was a tight muscle feeling as well as a particular sensitivity with the uppermost vertebra. The patent's job as a manicurist demanded that she keep her head turned for long periods during the day. The doctor, suspecting subluxation, performed diagnostic tests and proceeded with treatment. After a few weeks, the patient reported that her headache symptoms had substantially diminished. On a scale of 1 to 10, the patient rated her pain as a 4, while she had rated it a 10 before visiting the chiropractic doctor.

This case illustrates the central aim of chiropractic. A headache merely directs the doctor toward its root in the spinal column. By making precise corrections to the vertebrae, the nervous system is allowed coordinate the body's inborn healing mechanisms, thus abating the pain. This approach ensures that the chance of future attacks is also reduced.

Having outlined the chiropractic approach to health care, we may now turn to the specific causes and ramifications of back pain. In doing so, we take the first step toward understanding its prevention and treatment.

Cumulative and Single-Incident Injuries

Damage to the spinal column can result from a myriad of traumas. It may hit you after a long car ride or after sleeping in a bad position. It can happen after a bad fall. It may come from poor posture or crouching over your desk at work. Whatever the specific cause, back pain generally comes from trauma that is the result of accidental injuries, misuse, or unfavorable working conditions. Anything that puts stress on the spine jeopardizes your back. Stress may take the form of emotional strain or chemical stress such as alcohol, tobacco, or over-medication. The cause of pain can also be degenerative in nature. It can also result from seemingly small things such as unequal leg length. In short, an unbalanced spine is at risk. A change in the body's center of gravity can cause subluxation or damage to the disks.

For the most part, spinal stress is the result of a series of small traumas that build up over time. The term cumulative trauma is usually applied to repetitive strain injuries in the workplace. Here, we extend it to any accumulation of damage, such as habits that compromise the spine. As we have seen, any damage to the vertebrae or disks can have drastic consequences for the back and systems elsewhere in the body. In a very real sense, the spine bears the weight of living. Everything we do puts us at risk. Awareness of these dangers will help you avoid them. Furthermore, when a spine is healthy, it is more resilient to accidents when they do happen.

Bad Habits

Back pain is an effect. Finding its roots not only reveals anatomical problems, but also the behavior that caused them in the first place. Perhaps the most common cause of back pain is general misuse—habits that alter the natural curves of the spine or the integrity of the disks. We will therefore explore some of the most notorious activities that harm our spines.

Many patients who suffer from lower back pain possess a hyperlordosis, or a curving of the spine beyond its natural shape. When a person slouches, for example, the normal curve of the upper vertebrae is straightened out as the head is angled forward. People who are overweight or pregnant tend to develop this poor posture. It can also come from simply having poor abdominal muscles. Since the spine is called upon to support the weight of the body in this compromised position, the likelihood of damage is great. Mainly, the consequence of slouching is that the disks bulge backward and irritate the nerves emerging from the vertebrae. Certainly, a habitual sloucher is at tremendous risk for spinal damage.

Another consequence of slouching is that the fin-like bones at the back of each vertebra, the facet joints, can become irritated. Because the facet joints are encased in highly sensitive cartilage, tremendous pain can result from their misuse. When they are out of alignment—or are forced to bear too much weight from a hyperlordosis—the joints register this stress as pain. The pain from the facet joints can often rival that of a disk condition. Over time, repeated trauma can result in severe complications.

Consider the posture you are taking as you read this book. Are you bent over a desk? Are you holding it at eye level? If you are bending your head forward at all, you can imagine how holding that position for a long time will result in muscular or vertebral stress. Although I'm sure the author would like your undivided attention, it is often best to take a break from reading. Allowing the muscles to move in a different way lessens the possibility of damage.

If you're still with us, then we will move on to other bad habits that grind the spine. Another common cause of back pain is repetitive improper lifting. By the time we're adults, we've heard the dictum "lift with your legs" thousands of times. The reason for this is simple. When bending down without bending your knees, the spine becomes rounded, allowing the disks to bulge backward. It is, in this sense, an extreme form of slouching. Damage can happen to the spine after bending over to lift something one time. However, it is far more common to find damage done by a continued practice of improper lifting. This kind of cumulative damage is common with those who work in situations that demand repeated lifting, such as working in a warehouse. It is also important to avoid twisting when lifting.

The ultimate price of carelessness is debilitating back pain that may take weeks or months to heal. More than half of workman's compensation claims is the result of back injuries. This spells out a loss of wages and a reduced quality of life.

Another infamous source of back pain is repetitive strain from excessive twisting and turning during daily activities. A person working at a desk must turn regularly throughout the day to use items around the desk. This repeated motion puts stress on the disks, and especially the annular fibers surrounding the nucleus of each disk. These fibers can develop lesions when stressed in this way. The facet joints are also vulnerable to damage under these conditions.

If moving in the wrong way can cause damage, so can remaining in the same position. If the spine is in the flexed position too long—as when bending over—the disks can become strained. An example of the flexed position is when we bend over to take wet laundry out of the washer. As we have seen, this activity, if repeated, can inflict great damage on the spine. An even more common example of the flexed position is sitting. Although we often perceive sitting as a restful position, the pressure on the spine increases up to eleven times when we sit. Today, as people spend more time in front of a computer screen, it is important to understand this form of spinal damage.

Those who spend much time talking on the phone, especially at work, often tend to hold the receiver between the ear and shoulder. This position is detrimental to the shoulder as well as the neck and middle back.

Those who stand for much of the day also must remember that proper posture must be maintained. They should not stand with stiff knees or their spines arched backward. The toll of improper posture can be felt in extreme fatigue and, of course, back pain.

All these habits have one thing in common: imbalance. Any practice that throws the spinal column out of its normal shape can result in subluxation, disk damage, and most immediately, great pain. A bus driver, for example, complained of back pain. The examining doctor noted that the patient had a rather thick wallet, which he kept in his right back pocket. Because of the patient's job, he sat in one position for long periods. Although having a thick wallet is usually a good thing, it was detrimental in this case. Because of his wallet, the patient was sitting off balance. After thinning out his wallet, the pain lessened and eventually vanished.

Given the many ways that damage can be done, you may be reluctant to move at all. This is a valid concern, especially if you have already suffered from an injury. However, it is important to keep your muscles strong. Motion in itself doesn't cause damage, just incorrect motion. In subsequent chapters, we will outline the best practices and exercises to keep the spine healthily active, while minimizing dangerous motions.

Trigger Points

An important mechanism involved in back pain is the occurrence of trigger points. Trigger points are localized areas of tenderness in certain muscles in the back and hips. Pain caused by trigger points can be transferred from one region to another. For example, a trigger point on the hip may cause pain running down the leg. They may also occur independently. These areas of tenderness form when muscles contract, producing waste products such as histamine and lactic acid. These waste products irritate the muscles if not properly eliminated. Ordinarily, they are removed from the muscle as it contracts and relaxes. But as we move about in our daily activities, the back muscles are put through a rigorous workout. If these muscles are tensed for an extended period, they may develop trigger points.

Clearly, trigger points can present a great number of problems for the back itself. They can be deceiving, however, because trigger-point pain can be transferred to other regions. An assembly line worker, for example, may develop tension in his shoulder muscles from repetitive motions. The resulting trigger points can transfer pain along the arm to the thumb. While fixed working conditions are the most common cause of trigger points, they may also happen to active people. A tennis instructor, for example, may complain of back pain although she'd experienced no accident and was strong and healthy. Trigger points along her back may be causing the pain.

Subluxations may have a similar effect as trigger points. Although they are different ailments, a misalignment in the atlas vertebra (the vertebra connected directly to the base of the skull) can transfer pain to the lower back, legs, or shoulders. Both these sources of pain can be treated with careful adjustments or massage.

The Pain Cycle

Another concept important to understanding cumulative disorders is the pain cycle. As we have stated, pain is the body's signal that something is awry. Patients often experience back pain and associate it with muscle spasms. A muscle spasm, however, is a *response* to pain. When a disk or facet joint is damaged, a pain signal is sent to the brain. The brain responds to this by signaling the muscle to contract in an effort to prevent any damaging movement. When a muscle remains contracted for a long period, circulation to the area decreases. This in turn creates stiffness and pain, which generates more signals to the brain, and so on. An example of this can be felt if you clench your fist and hold your arm upward. Without fresh blood and oxygen, you begin to feel pain.

The lesson here is that motion is the key to health. When repetitive misuse causes trauma, the result is inflammation or muscular stiffness. Since motion is then limited, proper functioning is hindered and the area fails to receive proper nutrition. The weakened area is thus susceptible to joint disease, disk rupture, or subluxation. The spine should therefore be supported by strong muscles that are treated properly and maintained by regular exercise.

Muscles

Muscular problems are the source of much back pain. Because the spinal column is bound up within a complex of well-hidden joints and thick muscles, it is important to identify muscular disorders. When a patient does not respond to treatment, the culprit can often be a muscle. For example, pain in the lumbar region may be due to a spasm in the iliopsoas muscle. This muscle is located along the lower spine, running internally through the body to the femur. It is a significant muscle in the movement of the thigh and pelvis. Because of its inaccessibility, diagnosing and treating it is difficult. Patients are often unable to pinpoint the pain, describing it as a diffused ache.

However, when the examiner does find it, it is clear: tactile pressure will produce an extraordinarily searing pain in the region. An estimated 8 to 15 percent of patients with low back pain can trace part of it to this muscle. This condition serves as an example of the complexity and difficulty of back pain diagnosis. It emphasizes the importance of a precise and careful search for the root of pain.

Psychological Factors

Emotional stress can play a big role in back pain. The presence of the pain alone affects one's emotional state. Patients may seek treatments for months or years without relief, creating frustration and despair. This is especially true for those who suffer chronic back pain. Because of this apparently untenable situation, the patient may suffer from insomnia, irritability, depression, lack of appetite, or loss of concentration. The patient may feel alienated if the pain persists because others may feel it's in their head, or that they're not really trying to get better.

The resulting emotional distress may turn back on the patient, aggravating the symptoms further. The muscular tension associated with mental stress can, as we have seen, set up a cycle of pain. The situation therefore becomes apparently insoluble. With a negative outlook, the patient feels there can be no relief. This in itself makes it less likely that relief will be found. Furthermore, a patient with a positive outlook is much more likely to concentrate on healing rather than anger or frustration. It is therefore important that those close to the patient (and the patient) acknowledge the reality of the pain and develop a way of coping with it until it is lessened. It is important to have a clear idea of what you *can* do rather than what you feel is impossible.

Chronic Back Pain

Any back pain that continues three to six months or longer is considered chronic. Chronic lower back pain is often the result of repetitive strain injuries received at work. Pain can come as the result of trauma that accompanies the *hypermobility* of vertebrae. By this, we mean that a vertebra moves in different manner than the rest of the vertebrae. The spine is designed as a single, flexible unit. When individual sections deviate from these normal motions, damage may happen. Although a hypermobile segment has not yet become unstable (a greater degree of dislocation), it nevertheless causes muscle spasms and may result in trigger points that translate pain to other parts of the back. This is one cause of chronic back pain.

Workplace conditions are most commonly associated with chronic back pain. When workers move in certain repetitive ways, or are pushed beyond healthy limits, they run the risk of injury. Injury can result from performing tasks with too much speed, force or redundancy. Often, there is inadequate training, supervision, or aggressive competition among coworkers. Poorly designed equipment can also force workers to apply more force than is safe. As a result, the workers experience muscle strain, hyperlordosis, or stressed disks and facet joints.

When workers stoop to perform tasks, they put stress on the cervical (upper) spine. Because this region houses the nerves that control the upper extremities, malfunction can cause pain in the arms and hands. Often, these workers also get headaches. Computer operators, beauticians, assembly line workers, and many others put stress on their cervical spine every day. Over 14 million Americans seek treatment for headaches annually. Worldwide, more than 13,000 tons of aspirin are consumed every year, mostly for headaches. We have mentioned the dangers of an over-reliance on drugs. Sufferers of headaches often become dependent on drugs, and suffer from rebound headaches—that is those headaches that are aggravated by the medicine taken to relieve them.

How does cervical damage cause a headache? When there is a misalignment within the cervical region of the spine, the nerves associated with those vertebrae are disturbed and send confused signals to the brain, resulting in a headache. The blood vessels associated with this region of the spine are also affected, decreasing the flow of blood and worsening the headache. The types of headaches that patients experience can become severe. They may feel vertigo, nausea, and persistent, throbbing pain.

Since the nature of most back pain is cumulative, it applies to the daily, unceasing small damage the workplace presents. Much can be done through education of managers and workers. But when damage does happen, spinal adjustment is tremendously useful, especially in the relief of headaches originating from the upper spine. Today, adjustments can be done with great accuracy using specialized equipment.

As a brief footnote, it should be said that the highly stressful situations at work tend to worsen matters. When people are forced to work at a machine's pace, they are diminished not only in flesh, but in spirit as well. Discouragement, bitterness, and stress can have very real physical consequences.

Degenerative Disorders

Sometimes, back pain is caused by wear and tear. This is an unavoidable consequence of the passage of time. However, understanding the roots of degenerative conditions can help you to take measures to lessen their impact.

We consider first the degeneration of the disks. The annulus fibrosis, or elastic rings surrounding the nucleus of the disk, may wear out from stress. Twisting and shearing of the disks inflict trauma on them. If the resulting damage goes untreated for long periods, the outer wall of the disks can tear or bulge. The nerve roots passing near the disks may become irritated. In the most extreme cases, disks can rupture, letting the jelly-like nucleus of the disks ooze out and cause tremendous pain. Clearly, any damage to the disks can result in disaster if allowed to degenerate this far.

Bone spurs, or calcium-build up around the vertebrae, can also cause great pain when they irritate the nearby nerves.

Degeneration of the spine as the result of untreated subluxations or other damage can be put into a set of stages. A healthy spine—where the curves are gentle and disk spaces are even—can handle physical stress and has a full range of motion. However, as we age, with subluxations present spinal degeneration begins:

Phase I (birth to age 20)

> Loss of normal spinal curve.
>
> Disk, join, muscle, and nerve damage.
>
> Posture is distorted.
>
> Less physical energy.
>
> Height may diminish.

Phase II (ages 20 to 40)

> Increased decay, disk narrowing and bone deformation.
>
> Spinal canal narrowing.

Aches and pains more common.

Fatigue.

Reduced ability to cope with stress.

Height decreases further.

Phase III (ages 40 to 65)

Greater posture imbalance.

Increased nerve damage.

Permanent scar tissue.

Advanced bone deformation.

Beginnings of physical or mental weakness.

Phase IV (ages 65 and older)

Degeneration of cartilage and bone.

Bone fusion, constant pain and discomfort.

Increased loss of height.

Severely limited range of motion.

In general, the worse conditions are those that show severely decayed vertebrae. When calcium build-up progresses to the point of fusing the vertebrae together, serious health problems result. In an advanced degeneration, the facet joints are unaligned, resulting in great pain. Subluxations are more likely then, too. Spinal adjustment can reduce or even halt spinal degeneration by improving spinal posture and balance, thus keeping the nerves, disks, and joints strong.

Whiplash

We saved the most glamorous source of pain for last. Whiplash, simply defined, is acute neck pain as the result of a single accident. In this sense, it is similar to any such injury resulting from a sudden force on the spine, such as falling from a tree. Symptoms of whiplash are:

- Back and neck pain.
- Headache.
- Dizziness.
- Blurred vision.
- Ringing in the ears.
- Numbness in arms or face.
- Neck stiffness.

A rear end collision is the most common source of whiplash. The violent jarring places 12 to 16 g's of force on the neck (12 to 16 times the force of gravity) in a period of only a few seconds. Eighty percent of injuries from rear impacts occur at speeds of 6 to 12 miles per hour.

In the 1960s, whiplash was said to be the result of the neck being suddenly extended beyond its limits. This causes a tearing of muscles and ligaments as well as lesions to the disks. Recent researchers, however, contend that muscles are resilient enough to sustain this kind of damage, and would not result in such pain. They contend that much of the damage is not the result of over-extension of the neck, but rather a far less dramatic motion that nevertheless strains the facet joints and disks. Evidence also exists that concussions occur during collision. In any case, the structures of the vertebrae and disks are assaulted, causing pain.

Studies have shown that only 12% of whiplash injuries are well after a ten-year follow-up report. To be effective, treatment must be given soon after the injury, within two years, since symptoms are unchanged after that.

Summary

Having seen various causes of back pain, we can appreciate how spinal adjustments can address the roots of it, rather than just palliate the symptoms. Precise adjustments allow the body's inborn healing ability to restore health to the spine. By making sure the spinal column is balanced, through exercise or treatment, the body is more resilient. While accidents happen, a healthier spine is much more likely to heal or bounce back than an unhealthy spine.

We have seen that back pain is the result of the many stresses we put on our backs. We have also seen that most disorders are the result of habitual misuse, the accumulated trauma over time. Understanding this minefield of possible injury makes us more likely to avoid situations that put the spine at risk. Chronic pain can set in motion psychological stress that can, in turn, aggravate the pain further. Emotional encouragement and a positive outlook are important weapons against back pain. With careful prevention, precise diagnosis and treatment, a solution to the costly epidemic of back pain—though a formidable and complex task—is within our reach.

Chapter 3

Preventing Back Pain

Introduction

A patient complains to a doctor: "Doctor, it hurts when I do this."

Doctor: "Then don't do that."

Simplistic, silly and trite as it is, the advice in this old joke is inherent to any discussion of back pain. For instance, since bending at the waist stresses the spine, it should be implicit that to avoid back pain, you should not lift this way. This does not mean, of course, that we should never move at all. It simply means that we should move in the right way. What is the difference between the right and the wrong way? Most of the time, common sense will tell you: if it hurts, then don't do it. On the other hand, there is no substitute for good advice because many sources of back pain are not so apparent. Talking explicitly about it helps to raise concerns that we may not have considered.

We have already seen the statistics:

- 80% of Americans suffering back pain at least once.
- $50 to $75 billion spent on back pain.
- Fifty percent of workmen's compensation focused on the lower back, with well over one million workdays lost to back pain.

It is a perilous world. But does this mean that we simply resign ourselves to this peril? Should we push ourselves headlong through it, hoping that we can mend our ills after they have happened? Surely, it is wiser to avoid as many of them as possible.

In this vein, then, we must explore methods of steering clear of back pain pitfalls. We will present some specific tips for strengthening your back in order to help reduce the likelihood of damage. This will help underscore one of the main tenets of chiropractic: i.e., a healthy spine is less likely to suffer injury.

Good Advice

Mention the word "advice" to some, and they immediately think of unwelcome attempts to convince them of ideas that have no value to anyone but the advice giver. Those with back pain are frequently deluged with such advice, compounding their physical pain with frustration. Further, the flood of advice for *treating* back pain is rivaled only by advice for *preventing* it. Much of it is useful while much is ineffective, or even harmful. In the end, it comes down to personal judgement. In weighing the evidence, it is important to consider the variety of opinions and adopt those that suit you. Advice givers usually mean well and intend the best. We will therefore look at advice that has produced the best results and has stood the test of time.

Posture

We begin with posture because it suffers from the mother syndrome. The admonition offered (stereotypically) by your mother to "stand up straight" is ineffective by itself. It may even aggravate matters, since it reduces the advice to nagging, which we tend to either ignore or defy. As we grow up, then, many of us make slouching a full-time habit, and rarely consider standing up straight. As adults, however, we can recognize objectively the importance of posture. The first step to correcting faulty posture is to understand how it causes damage. The second step can simply mean making an effort to stand straighter. It can also mean strengthening the back muscles to be able to maintain proper posture.

If the vertebrae were stacked perfectly straight, there would be fewer back problems. However, since the spine is designed to curve like an S, the center of gravity is delicately balanced. Any deviation from that center results in abnormal spinal curves that can damage the vertebrae, disks, or muscles. Imagine the spine as a stack of checkers. A straight column has great stability. If the column curves a little, they begin to waver a bit. If you press your thumb on the top checker, an unstable column will burst apart, sending the checkers everywhere. While your vertebrae do not typically fly across the room, they nevertheless suffer stresses that, when continued uncorrected, can inflict harm. Since the spine differs from the checker column in shape, it must maintain its center of gravity in a curved position. This makes it vulnerable.

In terms of posture, the neck vertebrae are especially vulnerable. Because the human head weighs on the average 10 pounds, the neck vertebrae in a normal posture will bear that much weight. For someone who slouches forward, however, the neck vertebrae must support up to 20 pounds. We can understand, therefore, how an extreme hyperlordosis can cause the disks to bulge backward, irritating nerve roots or facet joints. It can make disks vulnerable to rupture and loss of flexibility. Reduced flexibility means the back muscles are less able to function within normal range of motion. Muscle spasms can cause a tightening reflex, which causes more spasms, and thus more reflex. Compounding this cycle of pain is the formation of trigger points, which can transfer a localized pain to other regions.

All this is to say that poor posture can have some significant consequences. Prolonged bad posture has even greater consequences. And so, an important prerequisite for curing back pain is making sure the spine is in a position that will retain the proper curvature.

Your spine should be shaped like a lazy S. Slouching forward will stress it. Standing too erect, as in a military posture, can stress the lower curve as well. To find the correct posture, stand one foot away from a wall. Lean against the wall, bending your knees slightly. Tighten your abdominal and buttock muscles, tilting the pelvis backward and flattening the lower spine. Holding this position, inch up the wall to standing position by straightening the legs. Now walk around the room with that posture. Place your back against the wall again to see if you have maintained it.

Good posture, no matter how you achieve it, is important in preventing back pain. There is no cure-all for bad posture habits. It lies in the realm of behavior modification. Because we form habits when we are young, it is best to encourage healthy activity for children, who imitate what they see in adults around them. For adults, since it is very difficult to change posture once the habit is formed, it takes perseverance. There are programs available for modifying posture habits. But at the very least, it takes simple awareness. The exercises discussed later in this chapter will also help to strengthen the muscles that maintain posture.

Lose Weight

Being overweight puts a tremendous amount of stress on the back. A heavy person's spine is distorted beyond its normal curvature. Further, the weight placed on this spine makes back pain much more likely through disk bulging, facet joint irritation and nerve interference. This imbalance can wreak havoc with the nervous system, resulting in serious conditions elsewhere in the body. Imagine it this way: if you are fifteen pounds overweight, it is like carrying a fifteen-pound bag with you at all times. Imagine how much easier it would be on your back if you didn't have that weight. It stands to reason that losing weight will greatly improve the condition of your spine, reducing the likelihood of serious back pain.

It is difficult to pick out the best weight-loss advice in a society flooded with self-help books and fad diets. These diets tend to promise quick results, but fall short of affecting permanent change. Studies have shown that 95 percent of people who use weight-loss diets will gain some or all of the weight back.

What can you do, then, to lose weight? Perhaps the best way to approach it is by seeing it not as a one-time activity of dropping a certain number of pounds, but as a permanent lifestyle change. The most successful diets are those that reflect a new attitude toward food and exercise. Diets often fail because we see them as a test of will power, to deny ourselves of those foods we love. This approach is ineffective because as soon as we feel denied something, we crave it, and eventually give in. Sometimes we revert to bad eating habits gradually, or in one large binge. But once it happens, we feel guilty or weak, and give up. We then re-gain weight and soon begin to diet again.

This "yo-yo" dieting can have drastic consequences to the body: when we lose weight, we lose muscle and fat, but re-gaining the weight, we gain back mostly fat. The result is a lowered metabolism, which means we are less able to burn fat. With each diet, then, it becomes harder and harder to lose weight.

Discouraged yet? Don't be. Discouragement, which often follows a single lapse in a diet, can lead to feelings of failure and depression. This is lethal to any program, and much of the reason that quick-fix diets fail. You should remember that losing weight is very difficult thing for millions of people. Further, good eating habits and exercise can *easily* be resumed, even after a lapse. A good attitude is your best ally.

Abandon the idea that losing weight will entail a few months of eating better. It will require a lasting revision of your exercise and eating habits. Gradual, realistic weight loss should be your goal. You should lose one or two pounds a week. It is also important to work with your health care professional to devise a plan that suits your own needs and desires. You will be more likely to follow a plan that allows you to take enjoyment from eating while doing it sensibly. Also, find the time of day when you will be most likely to fulfill your exercise goals, preferably a time when you've found it difficult not to over-eat.

At the risk of drowning the reader with advice, the following tips are useful in managing weight:

- Educate yourself on the best kinds of foods to eat. This may seem obvious, but it is sometimes forgotten. The knowledge you'll gain is indispensable. It will help you see through many of the quick-fix programs.
- Take it slow. A gradual change is more likely to take root.

- Do not starve yourself. This will only make you want to binge, and will make your body less likely to give up its fat in a self-preservation reflex.
- Substitute high-fat foods for lower-calorie foods, such as carbonated water or yogurt instead of soda and ice cream. Every calorie counts. Gradually step down your intake wherever possible.
- Do not shop for groceries while hungry. You will be more likely to buy impulse items, which usually means junk food.
- Read labels carefully. Calories are based on serving sizes that may are smaller than many of us realize. We also tend to eat more of low fat items because we feel there is more elbowroom in our calorie allotment. Many people therefore gain weight from these low fat foods.
- Eat slower. This will give your body a few minutes to feel full, and you won't over-eat.
- Keep a record for a few days of everything you eat and the amount of calories for each item. This will help illustrate your intake, and help you adjust your habits once you have become familiar with the calorie amounts.
- Tell your friends and family of your goals. Their support can go a long way in reminding you if you begin to revert.

In short: don't "diet." Eat better, move more, and do this for the rest of your life. By setting realistic goals and taking responsibility for a life-long change, you can lose weight and take the pressure off your spine.

On the Job

We now turn to the most familiar arena of back pain: work-related injuries. In workers under the age of 45, back pain is the number one cause of disability. More than half of workmen's compensation is paid for injuries to the back. Clearly, the stakes for industry are high. But while 90 percent of the money spent on back pain goes toward treatment, only 3 percent goes toward preventative or educational programs. As we have seen, most back problems occur gradually, from long-term, incremental damage. Disks wear out from repeated trauma, resulting in a bulge or rupture. Trigger points form, referring pain along the back. The chances of subluxations increase, putting the nerve roots at risk for irritation. The highly sensitive facet joints are also at risk under these stressful conditions. The following tips can help guard against the many perils in the workplace.

Lifting is perhaps the most notorious activity for causing back pain. At jobs that require frequent lifting, always face the object you want to lift and always keep the weight close to the body. An object held close to the spine's center of gravity will exert only that much weight on the vertebrae. Holding it away from you can increase this weight by as much as ten times. In lifting, straddle the object first. When bending over, even for a light object, it is important not to bend at the waist. Crouch close to the object while keeping your back as straight as possible and stand up keeping the same posture. You will feel pressure in your thighs as they flex to lift. This means you are lifting properly. Any lifting practice that makes the spine droop forward will severely stress the vertebrae and disks.

When lifting, it is crucial, too, that you never twist while carrying an object. Warehouse workers who frequently load boxes onto trucks are especially prone to this situation. The best way to do it is by holding the object as close to your center of gravity as possible. Then, take an extra step and turn your entire body without twisting at the waist. This may seem robotic and slow, but it will save you from back pain and lost work.

Another tip important to lifting is that when an object is very heavy or awkward, get help if possible. No one will be impressed if you lift an enormous bulk and throw your back out. Your boss, especially, will be unamused if you try something foolish for the sake of time.

Some warehouse workers, or anyone who lifts frequently, use a brace that adds support to the back. These can be of great value and come highly recommended.

While we're on the subject of lifting, consider a technique that can be used in any part of your life, whether lifting boxes at work or laundry at home: the tripod lift. To do this, simply get down on one knee, slide the object up the leg that is on the ground and onto the other thigh. Then stand, using the muscles in your legs while keeping the object close to your body. Another good technique is called the "golfer's lift," named after golfers who take the ball from the cup while balancing their weight on their putter. When bending in this fashion, the only motion is at the hip as you keep your spine straight and balance yourself on an object—a chair or cabinet door. The key to both of these methods is maintaining the normal shape of the spine while lifting.

If your job entails working in an office, there are many risks you should consider. Repetitive strain disorders require just that—repetition of motion. Although objects around the office are not heavy, the frequency of certain activities inflicts cumulative injuries on the spine. Injury may come from staying in one position too long as well.

At the office, the great danger is slouching while at the desk. To avoid putting strain on the lower back and neck vertebrae, sit at your desk with your buttocks flat against the back of the chair, with feet flat on the floor. The knees and elbows should bent be at a comfortable 90 degrees. Put the height of the chair at a level that doesn't require bending over. If you have a chance, stand up for a few minutes every hour or two to relieve stress on the lower back. You can also use a cushion for your lower back to ease the weight of sitting for long periods. Remember that when sitting, there is greater stress on the spine than when standing.

Make your environment work for you. Arrange objects around your desk so that you don't have to twist to reach them. You shouldn't have to move your head too much to do your work. Your computer screen should be placed directly in front of you, with the top of the monitor at eye level. Keeping your head bent forward as in reading causes your head to hang on your neck ligaments, spraining them. When talking on the phone, never cradle it between your shoulder and head, as it strains the neck vertebrae. Get a headset, speaker-phone, or simply get in the habit of holding it with your hand. Putting the neck vertebrae at constant risk will eventually catch up with you.

Standing positions, though they put less stress on the spine, can be harmful as well. If you stand with a straight posture, there is minimal pressure on the vertebrae. Any deviation from the center of gravity, however, puts you at risk. Since you are less restricted in movement when standing, there is greater likelihood of wavering. Try to retain the best posture you can. Every effort will help.

If your job entails standing for long periods, avoid wearing high heels, as this puts the pelvis into misalignment with the lower spine, causing it to compensate by bending beyond its range.

Try to prop one foot on a small stool when standing. This will take pressure off the lower back by restoring a healthy curve. Avoid "swayback," or standing with your knees locked backward and neck bent forward. This causes the spine to curve forward in the lumbar region while curving backward near the shoulder blades. Instead, stand with knees properly flexed forward. Strong abdominal muscles are helpful here.

All this advice stands for those working on the assembly line. Care should be taken when lifting as well as standing or sitting in one place for a long time. Avoid reaching for objects above your head. If you need to do overhead work, get a ladder or stool. Notify a supervisor if faulty equipment causes you to exert more force than should be required. Operating such equipment can cause serious strain to the lower back. Do not be over-competitive with your co-workers. This can lead to rapid and careless movements that when repeated over a workday can harm the ligaments, disks, and facet joints.

More and more employers are recognizing the dangers of repetitive strain and implement measures to reduce them. However, it is your back, and any condition at work that puts it at jeopardy should be taken seriously. Your spine is a vital part of your health and happiness. Employers who do not recognize this run the risk of losing you to back pain or bad morale. It is in their economic, if not humane interest to watch your back.

Sleeping

Because we spend a third of our lives sleeping, it is important to consider the position of the spine in this position. But before you can sleep, you must get into bed. Believe it or not, there is a right and a wrong way to get into bed. First, sit on the edge of the bed both arms to your side. Then, lower your body onto the side while keeping your legs at 45 degrees. Although it seems trivial, this action is repeated so often that it deserves attention. It is also especially helpful when you have back pain already and wish to minimize further damage.

In creating the best sleeping circumstances, you must choose proper equipment. Do not use hard foam-rubber pillows. These pillows force your head forward, stressing the neck. A pillow should support your head in a way that mimics the curve of your neck when you are standing with proper posture. Conversely, if the pillow is too thin or if you sleep without one, the neck will be stressed downward when sleeping on your side. Some pillows are designed to fit the contour of the neck.

Your mattress should be firm but yielding. A contradiction? Not really: the pillow shouldn't be so hard that it causes loss of circulation and sleep, but not so soft that it will distort the spine. Your back needs support, but since it is naturally curved, an absolutely straight surface will compromise it as well. Find a balance. Since most mattresses are far too soft, you will probably need to get a firmer one. If a new mattress is economically unfeasible, then try putting a bed board (usually made of ¾ inch plywood) between your mattress and bedspring. Either way, if you have a bad mattress, you will not only stress your spine, but you will lose sleep—which, after all, is the point of a mattress in the first place.

Sleeping on your stomach stresses the neck vertebrae by twisting the neck. Try to sleep on your back, with your back straight and head in line with your spine. Your head should be pitched neither forward nor backward. If you sleep on your side, a small pillow between your legs will help align your hips. Do not sleep in an extreme fetal position, with your knees curled up to your chest, as it reverses the spinal curves excessively.

We must avoid these positions. However, when we are asleep, it is difficult to alter our behavior. In sleep, deliberate efforts are impossible. The best you can do is to fall asleep in a desirable position, and to feel *comfortable* in that position. If learn to feel comfortable in a proper position, you will be more likely to assume that position when asleep. Some have tried extreme measures to alter their sleeping positions, such as sewing large buttons on the front of their pajamas to avoid sleeping on their stomachs. Whatever method works for you, remember that the position you choose should allow you to get solid rest, as this is important to your health.

General Back-Saving Tips

The following list of tips will help you maintain the health of your spine in various aspects of your life.

- In the car, keep the seat close to the steering wheel to avoid bending forward. Your body should be no further than ten inches from the steering wheel.
- Long car rides or rough roads pose the danger of an accumulation of small shocks to the lower back, causing trauma.
- Getting in and out of the car, you should sit on the seat first with both feet on the ground, then swing your legs in.
- If your car seat is not firm, use a small pillow for your lumbar curve.
- The car seat should be tilted so your thighs are level, or your knees slightly higher than your hips.

- When traveling by plane or bus, do not carry unbalanced loads of luggage
- Travel light. Do not over-pack.
- If traveling by plane, relieve the tension of sitting in one posture by walking up and down the aisle for ten minutes every hour or so. If traveling by car, plan to stop and stretch your back regularly.
- In the bathroom, when you brush your teeth or shave, avoid leaning unsupported over the sink. Open a vanity door to rest a foot on the inside shelf or balance yourself with a free hand.
- Never watch television or read in bed with your head propped forward. This stresses the neck vertebrae.
- Do not sit in deep couches or soft chairs. Never flop into a seat, as this may strain the neck with a whiplash effect.
- Keep a positive outlook. A good attitude can ensure that you maintain good back habits, but may also increase biological resistance to trauma.
- Avoid carrying unbalanced loads of any kind.
- When you cough or sneeze, round your back and bend your knees slightly. Do not turn your head to sneeze. If you have to turn away, turn your entire body.
- When making the bed, do so from a kneeling position.
- Break the cycle of pain. When pain does occur, the muscles respond by tensing. This tensing causes further pain, which causes further tensing, and so on. This vicious cycle of spasm-reflex can make the episode of back pain seem infinite. Through techniques such as massage, traction, or precise vertebral adjustments, this cycle can be broken, allowing the body to re-adjust itself to a healthy balance. Through careful maintenance of the spine, you can avoid getting into the pain cycle in the first place.

Strengthening Exercises

Regular exercise is a formidable enemy to back pain. Stretching and strengthening the muscles in your back helps reduce wear and tear on your spine. A physical fitness program can make your back capable of handling the unforeseeable stresses that will assault it during your life. While traditional exercises such as sit-ups, push-ups, or weight training are useful in strengthening muscles, you may wish to exploit the benefits of routines that are designed specifically to strengthen the muscles that influence back pain.

Always check with a health care professional before embarking on an exercise program. Some exercises may be harmful to those with certain conditions. This does mean that these people are excused from exercise; it means only that they must adapt the exercises to fit their personal level of fitness. People with osteoporosis, for example, can use modified exercises that help prevent additional fractures. Even for people with no serious condition, it is best to proceed with caution. But it is also important to *proceed*. The following exercises are meant to strengthen the muscles and tendons that support the spine directly or indirectly.

Another quick note: no exercise program can work unless it is practiced. Whether the program seeks to strengthen back muscles or lose weight, it hinges on the level of commitment. Find a way to enjoy these exercises: listen to good music or catch up on the news—anything that helps make it less of a chore. They may be boring, but the results are not boring. Soon, your feeling of good health will become its own incentive. Ultimately, the habit of healthy exercise will take on its own momentum, and it will become easier as you feel better.

The Routine

The following program should be performed twice daily, taking less than fifteen minutes each time. These exercises, combined with aerobic exercises, proper nutrition, and good posture habits can dramatically improve your flexibility and overall health. The program should be started slowly, with an emphasis on maintaining control over the motions. If any exercise is painful, omit it from the routine. You may repeat any move as many times as desired.

1) *Hamstring stretch:* Lie on your back with knees slightly bent. Pull one knee toward your chest until you feel the hamstring stretch. Hold for 10 seconds before returning to the starting position. Repeat stretch with the other leg.

2) *Adductor stretch:* Lying on your back, bend your knees and bring the soles of your feet together. Allow your knees to lower toward the floor until you feel a stretching in the adductors (the leg muscles that pull the legs toward the body rather than away). Hold this position for 10 seconds.

3) *Back press:* Lie on your back with your hands clasped behind your head. Tighten the buttock and abdominal muscles at the same time. Flatten your lower back to the floor. Hold this position for 10 seconds, breathing normally.

4) *Hip stretch:* Lie on your back with your knees bent, feet flat on the floor and hands clasped behind your head. Cross your right leg over the left knee. Keeping your head and upper back flat, roll your hips to the right until you feel the right hip stretch. Hold for 10 seconds and return to starting position. Cross left leg over the right knee and repeat.

5) *Two knee stretch:* Lie on your back with knees slightly bent. Bring both knees toward the chest and pull both knees with your hands, raising your head off the floor. Hold for 10 seconds and return to starting position.

6) *Head to toe stretch*: Lie on your back with knees slightly bent. Bring your arms over your head to the floor and point your feet down, away from your body. Stretch and hold for 10 seconds and then relax.

7) *Pelvic lift:* Lie on your back with your knees bent and your feet flat on the floor. Tighten the buttock and abdomen muscles together. Slowly raise your buttocks off the floor 4 to 6 inches. Hold for 2 seconds. Slowly lower the buttocks and repeat.

8) *Low back press:* Lie on your back with your knees bent and your feet flat on the floor. Tighten the buttock and abdomen muscles together. Press the lower back to the floor and hold for 10 seconds while breathing normally.

9) *Quadraceps press:* Lie on your back with your knees slightly bent. Place your palms against the right knee and raise the knee toward the chest while applying resistance with your arms. Lower the leg and repeat with the other leg.

10) *Pelvic crunch:* Lie on your back with knees bent and arms crossed over chest. Flatten the lower back to the floor. Tuck your chin to your chest and curl up, raising your head and shoulders off the floor. Hold for 2 seconds and return to starting position.

11) *Abdominal reach:* Lie on your back with knees bent and arms at your side. Flatten lower back against the floor and raise hands above and beyond the head. Slowly curl head and shoulders off the floor and reach upward. Hold for 2 seconds and then return to starting position.

12) *Hip roll:* Lie on back with knees bet and feet flat on floor. Take a breath and slowly exhale while gently rolling both knees to the right until both hips are off the floor. Return to starting position and repeat to the left side.

13) *Hip slide:* Lie on your left side with your knees and hips bent and head resting on the arm. Slide right knee upward and toward chest. Extend right leg until it is straight. Return to starting position and repeat the procedure on your right side.

14) *Leg scissors:* Lie on the right side with head resting on hand and legs at a slight bend. Raise right leg toward ceiling, keeping the leg

straight. Lower your leg to starting position and repeat. After set is complete, turn to left side and repeat.

15) *Modified pushup:* Lie on the floor face down with hands placed at shoulder level, palms down. Take a breath and slowly exhale as you push your upper body off the floor, arching your lower back. Hold for 2 seconds and return to starting position. Repeat as desired.

16) *Low back extension:* Lie on floor face down. Clasp hands behind your back and take a breath in. Exhale and simultaneously raise head, chest, and legs off floor. Hold for 2 seconds and return to the floor.

17) *Pelvic tilt:* Come to an all fours position. Allow your abdomen to droop toward the floor and hold for 2 seconds. Then slowly roll back upwards, arching the back. Hold arch for 2 seconds and return to starting position.

18) *Shoulder shrug:* Come up to a standing position. Take a deep breath and lift simultaneously both shoulders upward toward the ears. Exhale slowly and lower both shoulders. Relax and then repeat.

19) *Forward press:* Place your palms on your forehead. Try to push your chin toward your chest while resisting forward motion with your hands. Hold for 5 seconds and then repeat.

20) *Backward press:* Clasp hands behind your head. Try to push head back, looking upward while resisting the motion with your hands. Hold this position for 5 seconds and then relax.

21) *Lateral press:* Place you right palm at the side of your head. Try to move your head toward the right, with your hand resisting. Hold position for 5 seconds and then relax. Repeat for the left side.

Your back will work hard for you when you give it regular attention. However, since this program is extensive, you may be unlikely to follow it completely. While we encourage you to practice the full program every day, doing *something* is better than doing *nothing.* In general, exercises that increase the strength of abdomen and back muscles (both upper and lower) will make you more able to resist injury. The following are alternative exercises that can be practiced throughout your day:

- To strengthen your muscles and increase flexibility, you may also choose to do some exercises throughout your day that can be done anywhere, even in public.
- Rotate shoulders, forward and back.
- Turn head slowly side to side.
- Watch an imaginary plane take off, just over your right shoulder. Stretch the neck, follow the plane as it moves up, around and down, disappearing behind the other shoulder. Repeat on the left side.
- At any pause in your day—waiting for an elevator to arrive or traffic light to change—pull in your abdominal muscles, tighten and hold for 8 seconds without breathing. Relax slowly. Increase the count gradually day after day. After a week or so, practice breathing normally with the abdomen flat and contracted. Do this sitting, standing, walking.
- Before getting out of bed in the morning, press your head hard against the pillow and hold for 6 seconds. This will not only strengthen your neck muscles, but will help you wake up in the morning.
- As you start preparing for your day, brushing your teeth or shaving, pull in your abdominal muscles and hold them as hard as you can. Get in the habit of starting your day with your stomach muscles held in.
- In the car, while waiting in traffic, grab the steering wheel at three and nine o'clock—that is, on either side of the wheel. Try to pull the wheel apart and hold it. Do the same, while pushing inward. While stopped in traffic, you can also push with your palms against the roof of the car. You can also push against your knees using the muscles in your forearms, chest and abdomen.

- While waiting for an elevator, put your toe against the bottom of a wall and push hard. You should feel it in your buttocks, abdomen and lower back.
- On the phone, you can grip the phone and squeeze hard. Also, while talking on the phone, stand astride a wastebasket with legs out straight, squeezing in against it using the muscles from your legs and hips.

Adjustments

Up to now, we have said little on vertebral adjustment since it is usually considered treatment rather than prevention. However, we should note that a doctor of chirpopractic can help encourage health in the body by ensuring that the nervous system is allowed to operate unimpaired. A spine free of subluxations is in proper balance, thus allowing the body's natural healing mechanisms to work. By monitoring the vertebral alignment, the doctor can evaluate your health. Some patients find that regular visits to a chiropractor can help improve energy, relieve tension, and help make their spine more balanced and able to handle stress. Patients often benefit from a single visit, but regular visits are even more helpful. Through precise measurements and adjustments, the vertebrae can be kept in a healthy alignment for a lifetime.

Summary

We have covered a great deal in this chapter. Perhaps the most important lesson we should extract is that the spine is like any other system in your body: since it becomes damaged mostly through every-day practices, we must take care of it. Like maintaining dental health with regular brushing, the back must be given daily attention and, sometimes, regular vertebral adjustments. While health care professionals are very adept at diagnosing and treating disorders, they cannot reverse years of neglect in a single visit. It is far better to be stronger in general than to patch things up later. Through simple awareness, we can make sure that we keep our backs out of harm's way.

Chapter 4

Managing Back Pain: Diagnosis and Treatment

Introduction

You've done it. You've thrown your back out. Perhaps you've been in a car wreck. Perhaps you simply turned your head quickly and couldn't turn it back. Despite all your efforts to maintain strong muscles and a healthy alignment of vertebrae, it has happened. What now? Realistically, you won't rush to the doctor at first, but you'll wait to see if the pain goes away. Since back pain usually resolves itself in time, most people do wait it out. However, the pain can sometimes last for weeks without significant improvement. Considering the loss of pay and mobility, you may wish to consider other options.

Assuming, then, that you've gone to a back specialist, the healing process will vary depending on the nature of the problem. But identification of the ailment invariably precedes any efforts to correct it. In order to gain an appreciation for this process, we will explore the two phases of spinal adjustment: diagnosis and treatment. In reading the following passages, it is important to note that each patient has the ultimate right to decide how to proceed with treatment. It is *your* back. A second opinion is always your right. Any health care professional will respect that right when offering treatment options.

We must also stress that the adjustments discussed in this chapter should only be attempted by a professional. Serious injury can result from an untrained attempt at spinal adjustment.

Diagnosis

The Examination

Since back pain is a complex condition, it is vital that doctors gain as much information as possible. A visit to a chiropractic doctor must therefore entail a detailed assessment of the patient's symptoms, personal health history, and examination results. As in any other health care profession, this information goes a long way toward designing treatment options. Each case is unique. But the approach to all back problems and associated nerve dysfunction must begin with a careful screening. This not only aids the doctor in pinpointing the problem, but also helps in flagging serious conditions such as cancer that may require a referral to another health care professional.

The doctor must therefore collect a great amount of data, including information on seemingly irrelevant topics. One patient, for example, may recall a car crash years ago that has since caused complications. Another may reveal a high level of mental stress that has worsened the symptoms. In any case, these bits of information are important pieces that contribute to an overall picture of a patient's health. Along with the information gleaned from the personal history, the doctor will assess the results of the physical examination and other tests. He or she will then offer a treatment strategy that best suits the patient.

Examining a patient can be divided into two stages: a subjective and objective examination. The subjective stage includes the interview with the patient to establish personal history and symptoms. The objective tests include range of motion, leg length, and skin temperature tests, among others. Both stages are vital to the process. However, the subjective phase is especially vulnerable to miscommunication, and demands unique attention.

Subjective Examination

In the interview, the doctor must take care to rephrase questions if necessary, showing patience and understanding. While the doctor must make an effort to be sympathetic, the patient in pain can sometimes become frustrated. It may seem to the patient that rephrasing means that the doctor doesn't understand. But the questioning isn't some attempt to wear you down like some criminal under a bare bulb in a police station. The doctor is merely trying to see things from your perspective. By describing the pain from many different angles, the patient forms a more complete and more objective representation of the pain. Giving in to frustration is understandable, but will only serve to muddle the portrait of your symptoms.

It is also difficult to achieve productive communication because words may mean different things for each person. One person may assume a question is directed toward a certain area when it isn't. This kind of miscommunication can happen without either person realizing it, but can have significant consequences.

Assuming the doctor and patient have achieved good communication, the first step is listening to the patient describe the symptoms. To help in this, objective criteria can be used, such as describing the pain level on a scale, or referring to an anatomical chart to describe the exact location of the pain. The doctor will follow each description with a question designed to elicit helpful information. A headache, for example, can mean different things to different people. It may mean tenseness between the eyes or a throbbing throughout the head. People also have different thresholds for pain.

After hearing the description of the symptoms, the doctor must find out how long they have lasted and what medications have been taken to relieve them. With a headache, for example, the patient may be taking a medication that *aggravates* rather than alleviates the symptoms. The history of any particular ailment aids the doctor in deducing its origin. Questions should also be asked to establish what activities worsen the pain. Perhaps a patient describes having low back pain when in bed, but after discussing it realizes that the symptoms last for the first few minutes after lying down. The pain may have therefore originated from the day's activities more than sleeping habits.

In forming a diagnosis, the doctor must also integrate information on the general health history of the patient. This can include family health history, but focuses mainly on the individual's history—factors such as the patient's working conditions, sleeping habits, and previous episodes of back pain. Smoking or drinking habits may have an effect on a patient's symptoms, as they introduce chemical stresses that may influence the nervous system. Recreational activities that stress the spine may come out in this part of the interview as well.

Objective Tests

While the subjective interview gives the doctor a foundation on which to build an understanding, much of the doctor's evaluation depends on the objective tests. Below are some of the most common objective tests performed.

Leg Length

In this test, the doctor measures the length of each leg. To ensure accuracy, a few readings are taken with the patient on their back. A difference in leg length can throw the spine out of balance, making it prone to subluxations or disk damage. An unbalanced spine that goes uncorrected may yield symptoms of low back pain, headaches, sciatica, and other problems. A research study revealed that 11% of the people studied had one leg ¼ inch shorter than the other one.

You can test for unequal leg length at home. It is a quick and simple way to find out if you are at risk for this kind of spinal imbalance, and may indicate that you may need to seek a professional evaluation. To test for leg length differences, put on hard-soled shoes and lie face up on a bed, with your feet over the edge. Your legs should be kept together, with arms resting easily at your side. Your head must be facing straight

down. Have someone hold your feet together and look at the soles of
your feet to see if they line up. If there is a difference, it could be a
source of back pain down the road.

What is done for unequal leg length? Precise chirporactic adjustments can help to restore normal leg length. Although each case has
to be evaluated on a case by case basis, a normalization of leg length
commonly occurs.

Patients have found great relief after being diagnosed and treated
for leg length difference. The condition also illustrates an important
concept in chiropractic: any imbalance can result in dysfunction of
the spine and nervous system. By correcting that imbalance, the doctor goes to the root of the problem. The symptoms, by consequence,
are eliminated. This can mean freedom from back pain as well as an
overall feeling of good health.

Range of Motion

A good indicator of spinal misalignment can be seen in tests that
establish the patient's level of flexibility. An extreme example would be
a patient who cannot turn his head. This can mean that the vertebrae
have locked together, reducing the neck's range of motion to immobility. More commonly, only extreme movements will cause a limiting
pain. Turning the head may allow the person to look almost entirely to
the right or left, but will be limited to a range between the points where
pain is felt. This range tells the chiropractic doctor much about the possible disorder in the neck.

In a flexion or flexibility test, the patient will be asked to go to the
limit of his or her range. When at the range limit, the doctor will apply
pressure on the crucial area. If pain is felt, then something is awry.
Even if there is no pain during a flexion test, the range may be severely
limited. Both conditions point to a possible misalignment. The doctor
takes careful note of the contour and flexibility of each vertebra as the
patient is put through the tests. The patient is asked to droop as far

forward and backward as possible, as well as from side to side. Similarly, when testing the neck vertebrae, the patient will bend his or her head forward, backward, and side to side.

Palpation

One indispensable and reliable diagnostic technique is palpation, or scanning the spine by hand to detect abnormalities. Subluxations may cause pain by irritating facet joints and may impinge the nervous system, thus hindering the body's natural healing mechanism. In an effort to detect deviations in the spinal alignment, the doctor will carefully feel the spine, compressing the soft tissue of the neck or back. If a problem exists, the patient will feel it immediately as pain and alert the doctor. The tenderness is rated on a scale of 1 to 4, helping the doctor understand the severity of the problem. This procedure is necessary to find the root of disorder. It is a precise technique that requires great training and experience. Without it, the diagnosis would suffer greatly.

Similar to palpation is trigger point diagnosis. While palpation is a specific technique used to diagnose spinal problems, it is akin to finding trigger points in the sense of being hands-on. Trigger points are areas of tense muscles in the back that frequently come from repetitive motion. These points are highly sensitive or painful to the touch and may transfer pain along the back and to the extremities.

Treating them can involve concentrated massage. However, treatment is best handled by flushing out the reason for their occurrence, which may reside in a work-related situation or a misalignment of the vertebrae. A professional is best suited for finding the root of the problem.

X-rays

X-raying is an important step in verifying the findings of other tests. It allows the doctor to determine exactly where the problem lies and how to proceed with a treatment. X-rays also help verify that treatments have been successful or if more adjustments are needed. X-rays can detect cancer, fractures, arthritis and some infections.

The use of x-rays in chiropractic is the result of efforts to make spinal adjustments more precise. The work of John D. Grostic, D.C. established a standard technique for evaluating the x-rays by measuring specific points that appear in the image. Although the Grostic measurements do not dictate an ideal position of the spine in themselves, they are a valuable way to assess the alignment of the skull in relation to a standard derived elsewhere.

CT and MRI Tests

While the tests discussed above are reliable and invaluable, some conditions might demand the use of other techniques. X-rays, for example, are unable to detect ruptured disks. However, a Computed Tomographic (CT) scan can detect ruptured or herniated disks in 75 percent of cases. It is also a more reliable way to detect cancer or fractures.

Another test that may be used is Magnetic Resonance Imaging, or MRI. Unlike x-rays or CT scans, MRI has no radiation exposure to the patient. Some problems may be found with MRI easier than with CT scans, but many times a combination of tests is in order.

Largely because of cost and efficiency concerns, MRI and CT scans are done sparingly, usually if other tests have not revealed anything, if simpler, or if a serious condition with a ruptured disk is suspected. They can both be done without admission to a hospital and have minimal risk. Like x-rays, they are important means to verify diagnoses and measure the effectiveness of treatments.

* * *

Treatment

Freedom from Back Pain

We have spoken a great deal about the causes, assessment, and prevention of back pain. But when people think of back pain, they ordinarily think of what to do once it has happened. If you have suffered an injury, you are interested in getting better, as soon as possible. You want to know what your options are.

Assuming, then, that you have undergone a series of diagnostic tests, what can you expect? After the doctor has gathered the necessary information on your back problem and has ruled out the possibility of serious conditions that would require referral to an M.D., he or she will discuss the results with you. If adjustments are considered a safe alternative, you will begin exploring possibilities of treatment. Therapies range from very specific techniques of spinal adjustment to at-home care and rehabilitation exercises. This variety stems from the complex causes of back pain and the demands that each individual presents. Treatment strategies vary, depending on severity of symptoms, age of the patient, or disabilities that might affect treatment strategies. Treatment times vary, too, depending on a variety of factors.

Overall, spinal adjustment and adjunctive therapies have yielded great satisfaction among patients. In a study of 240 patients who were totally disabled with chronic low back pain, 81 percent found significant improvement after 2 to 3 weeks of spinal adjustments. Over 40 million people visited a chiropractor in 1997, with surveys indicating a substantially higher satisfaction over traditional medicine.

Clearly, spinal adjustment can offer great benefits to those suffering back pain. Understanding the treatment options will make you more likely to take advantage of these. In the following pages, we will examine the treatments that have helped free millions of people from back pain.

Treating Back Pain at Home

Perhaps the most practical advice that a health care professional can give is what you can do on your own to ease your back pain. Since most of the healing process goes on outside a doctor's office, it only stands to reason that treating an injured back should lie mostly with the patient at home. This process speaks to the heart of spinal adjustment theory by allowing the body's inborn healing ability to work for the patient. Once this mechanism can operate freely, the patient must ensure that no further damage comes to the spine. In this vulnerable stage, there are some important things to keep in mind to help speed the healing process:

- Do not apply heat unless instructed by your doctor.
- Smoking and the use of caffeine may aggravate your problem.
- Do not take hot tub baths without first consulting your doctor.
- Do not walk up or down stairs unless absolutely necessary.
- Do not sleep on your stomach.
- Avoid carrying unbalanced loads.
- Always turn and face toward the object you want to lift.
- Use a bed board under your mattress for firmness.
- When sleeping on your side, keep a pillow between your legs. This will ease lower back pain and sciatica. If lying on your back, put the pillow under your knees.
- If you are fatigued or in pain during activity, rest.
- When moving about, do so in a deliberate and gentle way. Move like a zombie. Quick movements can put additional strain on your neck or back.
- Try to become active again as soon as the improvement of your symptoms will allow, or if your doctor recommends it. This will help keep your muscles strong.
- Do not lift heavy things.
- Use a long-handled shoehorn to put on your shoes.

- Eat out or have someone else cook. Cooking requires bending, lifting and twisting, all motions that will aggravate an injured back.
- Try eating from a countertop, as it is higher and doesn't require bending over.
- Do not sit in deep, soft chairs.
- Let someone else walk the dog, as the jerking motions can cause further pain.
- Try to always maintian a positive outlook.

Applying Heat and Cold

Another home treatment for back pain is heat and cold therapy. The following program can be effective in easing pain while recovering from an injury:

Ice therapy or *cryotherapy* is an important part of the rehabilitation process because it reduces the swelling of injured tissues, tightens ligaments that hold joints together, and reduces pain. Apply the ice (in a towel) directly to the painful area for 15 minutes every hour. Continue this routine for 6 consecutive hours. Rest for two hours. After completing the initial treatment, repeat the ice therapy every two waking hours.

After the pain has improved by 50%, and only with your doctor's approval, you can try the following routine:

- Apply ice (in a towel) for 15 minutes.
- Apply moist heat (in the form of a moistened towel) for 15 minutes.
- Reapply ice (in a towel) for 15 minutes.
- Apply moist heat for 15 minutes.
- Walk around for about 5 minutes to loosen up the back.
- Rest for an hour and then repeat.

When the pain has improved by 80%, and only with your doctor's approval, you can apply moist heat for 15 minutes, then ice for 15 minutes, then moist heat for 15 minutes. Walk for 10 minutes. Rest for one hour and then repeat.

It is important to note during this home treatment program that initial contact with the ice will be cold (of course), and will be followed by a tingling sensation, then a burning sensation, and then finally a numbness. These are normal reactions. However, do not leave the ice on for a period longer than 15 minutes, regardless of numbness, as this can cause frostbite.

Is Bed Rest Best?

For years, those with back pain were instructed to get as much bed rest as possible, sometimes up to weeks at a time. However, this has recently been shown to weaken muscle strength and prolong recovery. A vicious cycle results where the weakening muscle leads to more pain, which makes the patient want to rest more, and so on. It is now recommended that for cases of acute back pain, the patient should resume normal activity as soon as their recovery allows. The best alternative seems to be a compromise between immobility and moderate activity. If you are recovering from back pain, try to increase your movements gradually and steadily.

Extended bed rest has been shown to discourage a return to work. The longer an employee remains out of work, the less likely he or she will be to return. After three months of bed rest, the chances of returning to work *ever again* drop dramatically. Most of health care costs go toward the small percentage of people who become disabled.

Exercise Therapy

Many of the exercises discussed in chapter 3 may be used in conjunction with chiropractic management of low back pain. Special adaptations of these exercises are required for those recovering from an injury. If you want to begin an exercise regimen, discuss it with your health care practitioner. While it is important to remain active and keep your muscles strong, you don't want to inflict further injury. Be cautious, start slowly, and do not do an exercise if it causes significant pain.

If your doctor approves an exercise routine such as the one in this chapter, is a good idea to prepare your back for it: apply moist heat (a wet towel) for 10 minutes followed by 5 minutes of ice (a moist towel with an ice-bag on top of it). The exercises should be done on a firm surface such as the floor or a mat.

1) *Pelvic tilt.* While standing or lying down on a flat surface, tighten the abdominal and buttock muscles to flatten your back. Repeat this several times a day. Contract and relax the muscle about six times at each session, holding each contraction for 4 seconds.

2) *Pelvic lift.* Lie on your back with your knees flexed and your feet flat on the floor as close to the buttocks as possible. Keep the knees together. Tighten the muscles so as to flatten your low back against the floor. Slowly raise your hips up from the floor and hold for 4 seconds. Repeat 6 times. If you cannot raise your hips from the floor, merely tighten the belly, the abdominal and buttock muscles.

3) *Knee-Chest.* Lie on your back and draw your right knee up to the chest and pull it down against the chest. Do this for a slow count of 4 and repeat 6 times. Repeat with left knee. Relax between each stretch. Repeat with both knees drawn to the chest simultaneously.

After the acute pain has diminished, do the following exercises. If you feel pain in your low back upon coughing or sneezing, do not do them.

4)   *Hamstring stretch.* Lie flat on your back and raise the right leg straight upward without bending the knee. Place your hands behind the knee while keeping the knee straight. Pull the leg straight up so as to stretch the muscles behind your thigh. Repeat 6 times on the right leg and then do it on the left.

5)   *Abdominal Strengthening Exercises.* Lie on your back. Flex knees and place feet on floor close to buttocks. Either cross your arms or place hand behind the head to support the head and neck. Do the pelvic tilt from exercise 1. Then raise the shoulders from the floor by contracting the abdominal muscles. Relax the abdominal muscles and allow the shoulders to return to their resting position on the floor. Repeat this exercise as many times as possible, starting with as many repetitions as you can. When you can do about 50 repetitions, you have achieved good abdominal strength.

6)   *Low back strengthening.* Do this with doctor permission only. Lie flat on your stomach with arms along your side, palms down. Slowly raise your chest from the floor. Feel the muscles in the low back tighten. Hold the chest up from the floor for a slow count of 4 and slowly let it down. Rest between each session. Repeat 6 times.

7)   *Outer thigh strengthening.* Lie on your side. Turn your toes inward on the right foot. Lift leg upward as far as possible. Repeat 6 times on right and then 6 times on left. You will feel pulling in the outer thigh and pelvis.

8)   *Inner thigh strengthening.* Kneel on the floor. Extend your right leg as far to the side as possible, keeping the knee straight and the arch of the foot on the floor. Slide your foot along the floor until you feel the stretch of the muscles inside your thigh. Then lower the pelvis to add stretch to the inner thigh muscles. Do it

slowly and hold for a count of 4. Repeat 6 times on the right leg and then repeat with the left side. These muscles which are tight at the beginning will loosen and stretch with subsequent exercise sessions.

In general, exercise therapy helps re-pattern the muscles and ligaments that support the spine. The connective tissues surrounding the spine are slowly rehabilitated, thus allowing for proper posture and healthy nervous system function. It is an important mode of treatment because many patients with back pain often have scar tissue on the fibers and muscles that support the spine, changing their resiliency or elasticity. A healthy exercise regimen helps restore better tone to these damaged tissues. Be patient when looking for results. Since you usually damage your spine by small degrees, it will heal gradually too. The results of greater strength and flexibility will make you less likely to relapse.

Supplemental Treatments to Adjustment

Minor Therapies

Some methods of back pain include electro-muscle stimulation, ultrasound, and microcurrent therapy. Each of these can act as a supplement to another primary treatment. With *microcurrent therapy*, extremely small amounts of electrical current are used to help relieve pain in the soft tissues of the body. It seeks to enhance the healing process by mimicking the natural signals that occur in the body when it is trying to heal itself. The treatment uses such low current that the patient rarely feels it.

With *ultrasound*, the soft tissue regions are treated with high-frequency sound waves. Since they have such a high frequency, as much as a million vibrations a second, the waves penetrate deep into the body and create a heat response. The vibrations help break down the unhealthy accumulations of calcium and other hard tissue. Patients generally feel little more than a relaxing sensation below the skin, although the gel used to apply the device may initially feel cool. This treatment can be applied directly to the area of pain. The rise in temperature increases blood flow and relaxes muscle spasms, massages damaged tissue, and speeds healing.

While *electro-muscle stimulation* sounds like something from Frankenstein, it is merely a special form of electrical current directed at a specific area. Aimed especially at the muscles, it helps break the cycle of pain discussed earlier. Swelling in the soft tissues is reduced and muscles are strengthened. Administering the treatment yields a tingling sensation. It is recommended for cases where pain is accompanied by swelling and inflammation.

Intersegmental Traction

The idea of traction as a treatment for back pain is an old one. In this procedure, the patient lies face up on a table that has rollers beneath its surface. The rollers slowly travel the length of the spine, stretching the spinal joints. This increases the blood supply to the disks and increases their elasticity. This results in a better range of motion for the spine as a whole. Patients report a great relaxation with this treatment.

Adjustment

Adjustment and Chiropractic Theory

The primary treatment option open to chiropractors is, of course, vertebral adjustment. While traditional perceptions of chiropractic sometimes paint a questionable picture, this is merely a stereotype. The truth is that techniques in adjusting the spine have grown more and more precise in just the last few decades. Not only have diagnostic techniques improved, but treatment has seen many breakthroughs as well. The present state of the practice is one of specific gentle adjustment to the vertebrae.

To appreciate the importance of these adjustments, consider the basic thrust of chiropractic theory: When the spinal segments become unaligned, or when disks bulge or rupture, the malfunction registers as pain. Sometimes this pain shows up in areas far from the source, such as headaches or sciatica. The imbalance hinders the operation of the nervous system, which controls the entire body and its natural ability to heal itself. The chiropractic physician is an essential player in re-aligning the vertebrae to allow the spine to assume its natural shape. The nervous system is then allowed to coordinate bodily systems freely. Since the doctor has re-aligned the vertebrae, inflamed tissues are also able to heal.

This should be a familiar idea by now. It is an elegant notion, but daunting in practice. Because the spine is embedded within a complex structure of muscles and ligaments, the chiropractor must rely on as many sources of diagnosis and treatment as possible. However, the basic aim is always the same: align the vertebrae to let the body heal.

When the chiropractor implements a treatment plan, patients sometimes feel immediate relief. They sometimes feel discomfort while the body's systems acclimate to the change. But most patients respond favorably within a few weeks of chiropractic care. Some disorders take longer to heal than others. In any case, the treatment will probably be faster than traditional methods, and will yield greater patient satisfaction.

Upper Cervical Chiropractic

The role of the chiropractic physician is to find the least invasive way to let the body heal itself. To do this, the doctor must call upon the most accurate techniques available. The adjustment should be delivered only to the malfunctioning joint. Numerous techniques seek to correct a subluxated vertebra. Some of them entail slow, steady pressure while others require a sudden thrust. Some techniques traction to allow the vertebrae room to resume their natural arrangement. Sometimes, massage techniques are integrated. Always, the doctor aspires to precision.

Much of chiropractic is done with a broad spectrum of spinal adjustive techniques. Contrary to the limb-bending, joint-wrenching stereotype, most are extremely safe, effective and painless.

To live up to this ideal, Upper Cervical Chiropractors use special instruments to adjust the vertebrae. The purpose is to deliver a low-force thrust over a concentrated area. This allows the doctor to get right to the problem without disturbing other joints.

This device uses a movable arm that can be adjusted to deliver a thrust to the cervical vertebrae from any direction. Since the device moves in exact angles along many different planes, the doctor is granted a great amount of precision. A stylus makes contact with the vertebrae while a mechanical impulse is delivered with a controlled amount of force, which is regulated by the doctor. The force is gentle, sometimes imperceptible, but the results are dramatic. Take, for example, one patient who had been experiencing intense sciatica and low back pain. She had been to two other chiropractors and medical doctors to no avail. With one treatment using an Upper Cervical machine, the pain was eliminated. It is a simple but powerful treatment.

In all, chiropractic adjustment works to treat back pain because it improves mobility between vertebrae, thus reducing the inflammation that accompanies locked vertebral joints. This mobility relieves nerve irritation and allows the muscles surrounding the spine to relax, thus breaking the spasm/reflex cycle of pain. Adjustments may also relieve bulging disks and the associated nerve disturbance.

Summary

We have seen in this chapter how a patient may progress through diagnosis to treatment. It should be clear from looking at these techniques that chiropractic is built on the idea of precision. Great care is applied at each stage of the process, whether it's interviewing the patient or making a vertebral adjustment. This focus on treating the patient is what many find appealing about chiropractic. Patients experience satisfaction at being given such close and careful attention. This positive environment is not just an added bonus, it is important to the healing process because it helps the patient maintain an optimistic outlook.

In the concluding chapters, we will encapsulate the main notions of chiropractic discussed throughout the book. We hope to put them in a perspective that will help you appreciate chiropractic as a unique form of health care.

Chapter 5

Questions and Answers

Introduction

When you suffer from back pain, you suffer from frustration as well. Often, the uncertainty of your condition is what separates a merely aggravating situation from an unbearable one. To alleviate this uncertainty, specific answers are needed. This applies to those suffering from chronic back pain as well as those seeking to improve their overall health. Throughout this text, we have endeavored to present the information with as much clarity and precision as possible. In addressing the following questions, we use the same straightforward ideal. This chapter seeks to condense much of the information already presented, while offering new insights along the way. Armed with this information, those who suffer from back pain (and those who want to avoid it) will be able to assess spinal adjustment as a reliable method of health care.

* * *

What is chiropractic? The word means "done by hand," and was coined by its founder, D.D. Palmer. The term reflects its main tenet: that health can be restored without using drugs or surgery, but rather through a hands-on approach. Chiropractic seeks to re-align subluxations—vertebrae that have shifted from their natural position.

To some chiropractors, the term "subluxation" can mean a loss of function for any reason, rather than a full displacement. However, all chiropractors know how these malfunctions can affect the health of the body. That is, since all the functions of the body are channeled through the spinal cord, a spinal aberration can hinder the function of the central nervous system. This hinders the body's natural ability to heal itself. By restoring the spine to a healthy state, chiropractors seek to aid the natural healing mechanism of the body, and thus relieve pain. Pain, in itself, is merely the sign of a deeper problem. By correcting the root of the problem in the spine, the pain—whether in the back, shoulder, or head—will subside.

This is general chiropractic theory. Many chiropractors, however, are not so strict on these matters. That is, they mix in other ideas from other healing arts, including mainstream medicine. These "mixers" comprise the majority of chiropractors today. Another division, the "straights," adheres strictly to the doctrine of D.D. Palmer, contending that all disease has its origin of the spine. The mixers, while they hold the idea that many ailments can be traced to the spine, recognize other sources of disease as well. Mixers also promote treatments other than just adjustment of vertebrae, and are more likely to work with an M.D.

Despite these variations in philosophy, all chiropractors are concerned with back pain, and techniques to cure it. They are all concerned with keeping the spine in proper alignment and balance. Because the spine must bear the weight of the body, many problems arise when the spine is off balance, resulting in pain. All chiropractors seek to use noninvasive, drugless methods of healing that pain.

How did chiropractic originate? The idea of manipulating the spine goes back to ancient times, most notably with Hippocrates, the famous Greek physician born in 460 BC who wrote, "Look well to the spine for the cause of disease." However, chiropractic in the modern sense began in 1895 when D.D. Palmer adjusted the spine of a deaf janitor who subsequently regained his hearing. Palmer thereafter founded the practice of chiropractic, establishing the Palmer Chiropractic Institute in Davenport, Iowa. Palmer's son, B.J. Palmer, continued to develop the art of chiropractic further. In the first half of the twentieth century, the numbers of chiropractors grew slowly, but were limited by a lack of acceptance by mainstream medicine.

A turning point came in the late 1970s, when Dr. Chester Wilk and other chiropractors sued the American Medical Association (AMA) for trying to condemn and abolish chiropractic. By 1987, a federal judge ruled that the AMA must not interfere with the activities of chiropractors. Five years later, the AMA altered its policy to allow the referral of patients to chiropractors. Today, chiropractic is a widely accepted form of health care.

How many chiropractors are there in the U.S. today? According to the Federation of Chiropractic Licensing Board, the number of licensed chiropractors in 1998 was around 79,000. Another estimate puts the number at around 50,000. You can find out how many chiropractors practice in your state by contacting the FCLB.

Federation of Chiropractic Licensing Board
901 54th Avenue, #101
Greeley, CO 80634
(970) 356-3500
www.fclb.[RTF bookmark start: _Hlt472584911]o[RTF bookmark end: _Hlt472584911]rg

Is chiropractic unrecognized? No. Chiropractic is recognized as a helpful and valid system of health care. The Wilk case of the late 1970s was an important milestone for chiropractic because it won governmental approval and ushered in widespread acceptance. Many people are still unaware of chiropractic's standing because, in its early stages, it was plagued by unscrupulous practitioners. Critics ignore that all branches of health care, including mainstream medicine, also had their share of questionable members. In chiropractic today, however, that is no longer the case, since all 50 states require licensing for chiropractors.

Mainstream medicine is also working closer with chiropractors. Since more people are becoming aware of chiropractic's validity, they are taking advantage of its benefits. One estimate puts the number of Americans who visit chiropractors between 21 and 28 million people every year.

What are the limitations?

Some conditions do fall outside of the realm of adjustment. Some include fractures, bone cancer, tumors, etc.. These conditions preclude adjustment, and should be treated by an M.D.. Your chiropractor will be aware of any similar conditions that would exclude adjustment, and will make the necessary referrals when indicated..

How long does treatment normally take? The treatment time varies depending on the severity of your condition. Some ailments may require only a short treatment program while other more complicated conditions may require a longer program.

While some see chiropractors to correct a specific problem, many see chiropractors for regular adjustments over a period of years, in the same way you'd have checkups at the dentist or MD. Generally, the healthier your spine is, the less treatment you'll need.

Are x-rays necessary? X-rays help the chiropractor diagnose the condition with accuracy. They also help in picking up any serious conditions, such as a tumor or fracture that would preclude adjustment. The doctor must know that it is safe to proceed with treatment, and *how* to proceed with it. X-rays are therefore necessary to make sure the diagnosis is sound and if the treatment is safe. Your doctor will determine whether or not x rays are necessary in your particular case.

What is an MRI and CT scan? Are they risky? Both of these tests are done to detect serious problems that cannot be seen on x-rays, or are undetectable in any other way. Because of cost and efficiency, conventional diagnostic methods are usually tried before these tests are ordered.

A doctor may use a CT or Computed Tomographic scan to detect rupture or herniation of disks, a condition that does not show up on x-rays. This test also detects fractures, infections, or cancer better than x-rays. In this sense, they offer an advantage. However, the CT test is not perfect since it may occasionally indicate an abnormality when there the disk is actually normal. Like all tests, it offers simply another piece in a larger picture, and should be used in conjunction with other evidence in forming a diagnosis.

An MRI or Magnetic Resonance Imaging is a test used to detect ruptured disks with 90% accuracy. An MRI is more expensive than a CT scan, but does not use radiation, so the risks are lower. Both tests can be done without admission to a hospital, and are valuable pieces in the diagnostic puzzle.

How does Upper Cervical differ from standard chiropractic? There is no essential difference between this specialty and the rest of chiropractic, except that Upper Cervical Chiropractors focus their treatments to the top seven vertebrae, called the cervical region. They seek to align the skull at a right angle to the spine because a misalignment in that region is crucial to the organs controlled by that area of the spinal cord. Often, problems in the cervical spine can result in complications to other areas of the body.

Upper Cervical Chiropractors aspire, like all chiropractors, to precision. They therefore make extensive use of x-rays to detect imbalances. They also use special instrumentation to affect adjustments on the neck vertebrae. Adjustments done in this way are painless, without the need for strenuous manipulation.

What kind of education do D.C.s have? Most state licensing boards require the completion of a 4-year program in a chiropractic college, followed by 2 years of undergraduate degree in general education. Many chiropractors gain special degrees called "diplomates" that focus on a specific area such as sports medicine. In 1997, there were 16 accredited chiropractic colleges capable of granting the Doctor of Chiropractic degree. Areas studied under a chiropractic program include anatomy, physiology, pathology, bacteriology, psychiatry, biochemistry, public health, and many others. As in other health care fields, chiropractors are taught to be sympathetic to suffering and to help the patient heal.

Do D.C.s work in hospitals? For the most part, no. D.C.s generally form their own private practices. However, D.C.s have been gaining more privileges in hospitals. Perhaps this is a sign that chiropractors will work in conjunction with M.D.s to form a more comprehensive alliance of health care.

Do D.C.s believe in medicine and surgery? Yes and no. Some severely discourage the use of drugs while most acknowledge that it is a necessary measure at times. However, the core philosophy of chiropractors involves using a method of healing that does not use drugs or surgery. They believe in the natural healing ability of the body, and seek to facilitate this process with alignment of vertebrae. They believe that it is more economical, efficient, and less damaging to exploit the body's healing mechanism than to force foreign substances into the body, further complicating things. A survey done by the Agency for Health Care Policy and Research noted that people suffering back pain would prefer to try a more conservative treatment like chiropractic before trying drastic surgery or strong drugs.

Can I see a chiropractor and my regular M.D. at the same time? Yes. While there are conditions that preclude chiropractic adjustment, there is no reason that it should be mutually exclusive with mainstream medicine. Since many M.D.s are working with D.C.s in clinics and on research projects, the likelihood of conjunctive health care is increasing. In fact, many M.D.s see a chiropractor themselves. In an ideal world, the two fields of heath care would supplement and enhance each other.

If the body heals by itself, why are chiropractors needed? Vertebrae are thrown from alignment after cumulative or single-incident trauma.

Misalignment doesn't just happen spontaneously. While it is true that the body has tremendous self-healing capabilities (a tendency toward homeostasis), this healing mechanism is impaired when vertebrae are out of alignment. In order to help the healing process—a process coordinated through the nervous system—a chiropractor repairs the spinal dysfunction. While a vertebra *could* re-align itself, this is rather unlikely. Waiting for such an event would take a long time. The chiropractor becomes an agent to accelerate the healing process by re-aligning vertebrae. A person with back pain often starts feeling relief only after a few visits. In any case, it is a lot faster than just waiting for a miracle.

Can I adjust my own spine? No. You shouldn't try. Some cases of accidental adjustment have been reported, including one as far back as D.D. Palmer, when he slapped someone on the back with a book. However, it would be dangerous to try adjusting yourself or anyone you know. Only someone with the proper training and education can evaluate when an adjustment is safe and how to do the adjustment without causing injury.

What causes the sound of adjustment? The popping sound is caused by air rushing into a joint when it has been slightly displaced. While not all adjustments cause this sound, it does happen. An adjustment that causes this sound is painless.

Is it bad to crack your neck a lot? People with a fixed vertebra tend to turn their heads sharply, like cracking the knuckles, to relieve pressure in the joints of the neck. However, this relief is only temporarily. It may indicate that you have a serious imbalance, and does not actually serve to adjust the vertebrae. The habit may be a sign that you have a subluxation. Cracking your neck is harmful because it ignores the real problem. Further, it can, like any stress to the spine, cause damage if done frequently or forcefully.

Can I tell if I have a subluxation without seeing a chiropractor? Not always. A subluxation may be very apparent if extreme pain is felt. More commonly, a subluxation can exist for a long time without being felt.

Regular check-ups can help in detecting a misalignment that can cause trouble for you down the road.

What happens if I visit a chiropractor only once? Once is better than never. While regular visits can help you, any visit to a D.C. will be of enormous benefit for you, especially if you are recovering from an injury or healing low back pain. Many people have reported that regular visits help them feel more able to handle the stress inflicted on their backs every day.

Who can use chiropractic? Anyone with a spine can benefit from chiropractic. This includes people both young and old. Chiropractic adjustments have been given to infants to correct complications from traumatic births. Adjustments are given to the elderly when there is no other condition that would exclude adjustment. The chiropractic ideal of prevention and treating the cause of a problem can benefit everyone. A healthy spine can help the young avoid back pain, and help the old minimize the damage done by degeneration.

Can a person who has had back surgery have spinal adjustments? Yes, as long as any fractures are healed. Many times, symptoms return after having surgery to alleviate them. Facing the prospect of more surgery, the patient may turn to chiropractic. Often, chiropractic is successful in finding the cause of the problem and correcting it. Adjustments may help prevent the need for surgery, saving a great deal of time and money in the end. Your Doctor will determine whether or not an adjustment is recommended in your particular case.

Can chiropractors detect cancer or other diseases? Because chiropractors are usually considered *portal of entry* practitioners, they are qualified to detect serious conditions while they do not treat these ailments themselves. Tumors, for instance, are sometimes detectable on x-rays. While chiropractors do their best to ascertain if a serious condition exists, they focus on their specialty—namely, adjustments. This means that they do not pretend to be a catch-all for disease. They recommend seeing an M.D. or other practitioner if a condition persists. All chiropractors are concerned with healing, even if it means referral. Chiropractors may also order MRI tests or CT scans if necessary. Overall, a chiropractor will offer his or her best diagnosis and offer a treatment plan. The decision is up to you.

What about osteoporosis? Osteoporosis is the thinning of the bones through loss of minerals, mainly calcium. It is a natural consequence of aging, and is a common cause of back pain in women over 50. The "dowager's hump" often seen in elderly women is the result of osteoporosis. Those most at risk for osteoporosis are white women over 40 who have gone through menopause. You are also at risk if you smoke, do not have a regular exercise program, have had low calcium intake for years, or if it occurs heavily in your family. One of the great dangers of osteoporosis is that your bones are easily fractured.

Much attention has been given to osteoporosis because it may be preventable. By getting good nutrition, your bones will be thicker, and will be able to stand a little loss later in life. Strong muscles also help you reduce the likelihood of fracturing a bone. The chiropractic philosophy of prevention and maintaining optimal health is clearly applicable.

What causes back pain in general? Back pain is such a complex phenomenon, it cannot be reduced to one cause. Much of it unknown, what is termed "non-specific" back pain. Even so, much of it *is* understood. In general, it comes from trauma that can be the result of cumulative misuse or a single injury. Most of the back ailments come from bad habits—those habits that fail to respect the vulnerability of the spine. To reduce the likelihood of back pain, we must pay close attention to poor sleeping posture, lifting practices, or work conditions.

Pain can result from stress put on the sensitive fin-like bones along the spine, called facet joints. There can also be a straining of the disks between vertebrae, resulting in their bulging backward and irritating surrounding nerves. The disks can also become irritated, or, in extreme cases, rupture, allowing the jelly-like substance inside to ooze out. Subluxation, or the misalignment of vertebrae, is another common problem, one that chiropractors are greatly concerned with. These conditions most commonly result in simple back pain. They can also impinge the functioning of the spinal cord and central nervous system, wreaking havoc with the body's ability to function and heal. The cause of back pain can also be muscular in origin. For instance, trigger points, or localized areas of tenderness along the back, can not only cause back pain, but also transfer pain to other regions.

Why is back pain so unpredictable? It often seems that back pain comes out of the blue. Why? The answer lies in the complexity of the back's anatomy. The spine is built to be flexible and strong at the same time. It must protect the spinal cord while providing enough flexibility to sustain the thousand shocks we inflict upon it every day. To ensure proper support, the spine is embedded in a complex mass of muscles and ligaments. This complexity makes the possibility for injury that much greater. It also makes diagnosis and treatment a challenging task. The many soft tissues surrounding the spine make it vulnerable. Considering the vulnerability and complexity of the spine, sorting out the exact causes is often difficult for professionals. For non-professionals, it can seem even more unpredictable.

What is a slipped disk? A disk cannot really slip. This term is used only for simplicity's sake. Disks can tear, bulge, herniate, or rupture. As the result of stress—consistently bad posture or lifting incorrectly—the elastic fibers surrounding each disk can weaken and even bulge. A bulging disk can irritate nearby nerves and cause back pain. Also, the inner portion of the disk—the jelly-like nucleus—can burst through the outer wall. Treatment for these conditions involves adjustments or traction. These treatments allow the vertebrae to re-assume their natural position. Often, the best recommendation is to avoid this kind of trouble in the first place. A person can avoid a great amount of back pain through regular chiropractic check-ups, good exercise, and habits that respect the natural curves of the spine.

What is a pinched nerve? This is another slightly inaccurate term. An actual pinched nerve, where bone contacts with the nerve, is rare. More commonly, a nerve is irritated or stretched as the result of a vertebral malfunction. Treatment for this condition is similar to a bulging disk: adjustments and traction. This allows the swelling of soft tissues to go down and helps the body restore balance on its own.

Can chiropractic help with headaches? Yes. Some types of headaches are more responsive to chiropractic treatment than others. But many patients have found relief from chronic headaches with chiropractic adjustment. This success can be accounted for by the nerve discomfort relieved by adjustment as well as the freeing up of blood vessels leading to the brain. This illustrates the primary goal of chiropractic—that is, to seek out the root of the problem in the spine to allow the body to heal itself.

What is scoliosis? How is it treated? Scoliosis is an unnatural curvature of the spine from side to side. If viewed from the back, the spine should be straight. Deviations from this center can cause serious health problems. Usually, scoliosis is *congenital*, or present at birth. Other times, this disorder can develop later in life from an accident. When it develops as the result of trauma, scoliosis is called an *idiopathic* condition. Traditional approaches to treating both types of scoliosis involve braces or surgery. However, chiropractic has been successful with congenital scoliosis if it is detected early. Scoliosis appears in girls more often than boys, although it can appear in anyone as a child or young adult. The exact cause of scoliosis is unknown, though it is strongly suspected that heredity plays a large role. It often appears as unevenness in the shoulders or hips. If the condition goes undetected, it can worsen throughout the person's twenties. It is therefore important to be alert to the symptoms and to contact a health care professional for detection.

Can the weather affect joints and back pain? Sometimes, patients complain of joint discomfort when there are extreme weather conditions. This is a very real phenomenon. When joints are out of alignment, they build up tension or pressure in them. If there is a climatic condition of high atmospheric pressure and high humidity, the condition worsens. Patients feel a gradual increase in stiffness and pain in joints of their back as well as elsewhere in the body. Applying moist heat twice daily, as well as doing exercises for the back (outlined in chapters 3 and 4) can alleviate the pain that is associated with this phenomenon. If the pain persists, there may be another condition present, and you should visit your health care practitioner.

What can I do to lower the risk of back pain? The short answer to this is to avoid any motion that exaggerates the curves of the spine. Avoid any repetitive motion where the spine is in a compromised position, such as bending over a workstation. There are many ways to reduce the risk of back pain, but it usually comes down to being aware of the conditions that harm it. Once the risks are more clearly defined to us, we are more likely to avoid them. Some of the most common situations that harm the back are: sleeping positions, lifting practices, and work conditions. You will find that most back problems result from cumulative misuse.

To avoid these dangers, you should place the objects at your desk within easy reach to avoid twisting too often. Sometimes the smallest motion, repeated in just the right way can have a cumulative effect. Take stretch breaks when sitting for long periods. Don't slouch; stand up straight, with proper posture (though not excessively military). Do not lift anything, no matter how light, by bending at the waist. Your mattress should be firm, and your pillow at the right height to avoid pushing your head forward or letting it droop downward. Use a backboard under your mattress if necessary.

You may also begin an exercise regimen, with the approval of your health care practitioner, in order to strengthen your muscles and ligaments. This strength will make your back better able to handle the stresses it encounters every day.

Are there less time-consuming alternatives to a full exercise program? Any exercises will help as long as you get in the habit of doing them. Although more exercises would help strengthen you better, anything you can do is better than doing nothing at all. Therefore, take advantage of those pockets of time during your day. If you find yourself waiting in line, in traffic, or talking on the phone, you can use the time to your benefit by doing some simple stretches and exercises. Chapter 3 outlines some of these exercises.

If I have a back problem, I'm reluctant to move at all. Is it dangerous to move in this condition? If you are in severe pain, it may be best to minimize your movements. However, it is important to keep active as soon as your injury will allow. It has been found that keeping your muscles strong is important to your recovery. Find a compromise between idleness and activity. If you are too idle, your muscles will weaken and prolong your recovery, while too much activity could worsen your condition. If you are doing exercises to strengthen your back, proceed slowly and increase them gradually. After a time, you will find that exercises have become easier, and your back pain has subsided.

Is bed rest recommended? For years, patients were told to get plenty of rest, often over a period of weeks or months. But this treatment does not seem to hasten recovery. In fact, it may hinder recovery for the same reason discussed in the question above. When muscles go unused, they weaken. This can not only lengthen recovery, but can lead to further pain by making the back more vulnerable than it already is. This weakened condition causes more pain, and the pain encourages more idleness, setting up a destructive circle. It is therefore important to make realistic efforts at activity, as long as your doctor approves it, and it doesn't cause you further pain. A strong back will heal faster.

Is chiropractic similar to massage? While chiropractic sometimes concerns itself with the muscles surrounding the spine, it mainly focuses on how the nervous system functions in the face of skeletal abnormalities. Chiropractors, of course, encourage massage techniques to relax the patient's muscles, especially with the occurrence of trigger points. Muscular strength and flexibility certainly help recovery from back pain. Overall, however, chiropractic concerns itself with problems with vertebrae and disks.

I was told to see a psychiatrist for my back pain. Are they suggesting that it's all in my head? While this suggestion may put you off at first, it isn't intended to imply that you're symptoms are fake. Psychological stress and physical pain are related. If you are in pain, you are under psychological stress. Stress can cause muscular tension, which can result in immobility of the joints and trigger points, both of which can cause further pain. The resulting pain can cause more frustration, and hence more pain.

We have seen this circular pattern in other ailments, where dysfunction seems to feed on itself, creating a cycle of pain. It is important, therefore, to stop the psychological portion of this cycle whenever possible. Frustration is certainly understandable, but serves to worsen your condition. The suggestion of seeing a psychiatrist may help in dealing with the stress that has contributed to your back pain. Evidence also suggests that a person with an optimistic attitude will recover more quickly and thoroughly because they concentrate on healing more than anger or depression.

Psychological evaluation considers the patient as a whole, not just a collection of mechanical parts that have gone awry. In this sense, it is a more understanding suggestion than a cynical one. The suggestion reflects an appreciation of the interrelated nature of a person's emotional and physical well being.

Does insurance cover chiropractic? Yes. More and more companies are offering coverage for chiropractic treatments. This is part of the reason for chiropractic's growth over the last couple of decades. The amount of coverage varies with each company, and you should check your policy or contact a company representative.

Where can I find out more about chiropractic? One easy resource is a local chiropractor. While this may seem obvious to some, others may have reservations about approaching a doctor's office for no other reason than curiosity. Most chiropractors would be receptive to inquiries because they're excited about the process themselves. You certainly have nothing to lose by asking. They may have resources themselves or would know where to get them.

You can also exploit the information available from organizations. Simply writing to these organizations can get a good mass of information. These organizations also have good web sites listed below.

American Chiropractic Association
1701 Clarendon Blvd.
Arlington, VA 22209
1-800-368-3083
International Chiropractors Association
1110 North Glebe Rd. Suite 1000
Arlington, VA 22201
1-800-423-4690
World Chiropractic Alliance
2950 N. Dobson Rd. Suite 1
Chandler, AZ 85224-1802
1-800-347-1011

The Internet, while a vast resource, is sometimes unreliable because there are no restrictions or editorial requirements for publishing information there. Any research done on the Internet should be verified through other sources. You should be critical with information from any source, but it is especially true of the Internet. Be careful.

However, there are some easily accessed and trustworthy sites. They offer a convenient way to locate a chiropractor near you while giving you a good start on learning more about chiropractic in general. Some of these sites are:

- www.chiroweb.com
- www.amerchiro.org
- www.chiropractic.org
- www.palmer.edu

In addition to these sources, you may also look to your local library. Here are a few suggestions:

Rondberg, Terry. *Chiropractic First: The Fastest Growing Healthcare Choice...before Drugs or Surgery.* Publisher: Chiropractic Journal, 1996.

Strang, Virgil. *Essential Principles of Chiropractic.* Publisher: Palmer College of Chiropractic, 1987.

Wardwell, Walter, I. *Chiropractic: History and Evolution of a New Profession.* Publisher: Mosby-Year book, Inc., 1992.

Chapter 6

Afterward: The Benefits of Chiropractic

Introduction

A tremendous satisfaction comes from being able to bring a person out of pain. Some patients spend years going from practitioner to practitioner, fruitlessly searching for relief. When the weight of suffering is finally lifted, it is an extraordinary moment for any health care professional. This is the reason chiropractors, like all doctors, are in practice: to end pain.

As satisfying as this moment is for the doctor, it is more so for the patient. Chiropractic can offer a unique opportunity for this kind of satisfaction. Too often, patients become enmeshed in a cold and impersonal process of health care. Medical terms have become synonymous with impersonal things: sterile, antiseptic, and clinical. While this is certainly not true for millions of doctors, many patients have negative experiences with the overall system, ranging from merely inconvenient to exasperating. In addition to their physical suffering, they find themselves burdened by anger and frustration.

How, then, can we realize that moment of relief? One observer noted, "the secret in caring for the patient is in caring for the patient." Sometimes, in the shuffle, the patient is forgotten. It is therefore important for health care professionals to remember to care for the patient first—to listen, empathize, and discuss the situation carefully and honestly. Only this way can a doctor hope to meet the patient's satisfaction.

Patient Satisfaction

Observational studies have consistently found that patients receiving chiropractic care for back pain are more satisfied with chiropractic than traditional health care. Patient satisfaction with chiropractic is, by one estimate, 3 times greater than traditional health care methods. The exact reason for this is unknown. Part of the answer may lie in the experience patients have in a chiropractic facility. The design of offices, for instance, often allows patients to see what goes on behind the receptionist's desk. This is just a small way that the patient feels a sense of trust for the doctor. It shows a unique sensitivity that chiropractic has for the psychological needs of patients.

The relationship that forms between patient and doctor is an important part of the experience. Doctors of chiropractic are noted for spending more time talking to patients about their condition. Patients feel that it is easy to confide in a chiropractor. This open communication results in a clearer picture of the symptoms and therefore a more accurate diagnosis. Furthermore, since the doctor doing the interview is the same one who will do the treatment, patients avoid an unsettling transition to a second doctor. There is also an important psychological dimension to the physical contact involved in doing adjustments.

The Placebo Effect

Some have suggested that chiropractic's satisfaction comes from an elaborate placebo effect. The term "placebo effect" indicates a process that heals a condition not by any physiological means, but by exploiting the power of expectation. A placebo is a medication that has no intrinsic value, but exploits the power of suggestion. A sugar pill is a classic example. If such pills are given for a headache, the patient may find relief simply on the *expectation* of getting well. The simple act of doing something—often anything—makes the sickness seem less formidable, something that can be controlled. Action gives us hope. Sometimes, the hope is more effective than the action itself.

Some suggest that the placebo effect arises from the close relationship between chiropractor and patient. These critics also suggest that because vertebral adjustment demands a "laying on of hands," it is akin to faith healing. What these detractors ignore is that *all* healing arts are subject to the placebo effect. The very term *placebo* has its roots in medicine. Patients often have tremendous faith in modern science, with a placebo effect commensurate with this faith. All healing arts must therefore consider the placebo effect in assessing treatments. Chiropractic is no exception. However, neither are allopathy, osteopathy, acupuncture, and so on.

All healers should remember that the mind can have a significant effect over the body. While the placebo effect may seem to muddle the results of treatment, it can be seen as an advantage. The placebo effect can be an important ally to the healing arts, using the power of the mind to do much of the work of healing. On the other hand, it is also important to consider the possibility of a placebo effect when assessing the effectiveness of a treatment.

Effectiveness of Chiropractic

If one of the benefits of chiropractic is patient satisfaction, then what are some others? Certainly, the special relationship between doctor and patient yields a positive environment that encourages optimism, which can go a long way in healing pain. But how effective is the treatment itself? Here, we can turn to special agencies that have studied the effectiveness of chiropractic adjustment. What are their recommendations? The Agency for Health Care Policy and Research (AHCPR) said in 1994 said that chiropractic adjustments—along with exercise and early return to activity—are effective. They recommended adjustments over surgery based on risk and effectiveness factors. Patients suffering from acute low back pain recovered quicker under chiropractic care than any other treatment. Chiropractic was also identified as effective in treating neck ailments, whiplash, and tension or migraine headaches. The RAND Corporation conducted similar studies and published similar results.

Chiropractic has also been revealed as a safer treatment for back pain than surgery. In comparing the number of malpractice suits between chiropractic and mainstream medicine, we see that chiropractic has an extremely low rate. Furthermore, one estimate puts the risk of complications from neck adjustments at 7 for every 10 million adjustments and 1 for every 100 million adjustments for low back pain. Compare this to the risk of 32,000 complications in every10 million from anti-inflammatory drugs. Adjustments avoid unnecessary surgery and unproductive hospital stays. One estimate done by M.D.s stated that only 1% of back surgery is absolutely necessary, with 90% of back surgery deemed preventable. In short, chiropractic adjustment is safe and effective in healing back pain.

While more research on effectiveness of chiropractic is needed—and may soon be realized—we cannot deny the persuasiveness of experience. Many patients can attest to the benefits of chiropractic. With this, and other pieces of the puzzle, we begin to see chiropractic as a reliable, safe, and effective method to treat back pain.

Case Reports

To illustrate the benefits of chiropractic health care, we present a few cases of actual patients. As you read these cases, keep in mind that different people respond differently to treatment. Their successes are not intended to imply that anyone with these conditions will get the same results. Doctors of chiropractic, like all health care professionals, can make no guarantees. In general, chiropractic *does* offer a safe and effective alternative to drugs or surgery. These stories are presented to illustrate the very real successes that chiropractic sees every day.

1) *A 65 year-old male experienced acute low back pain and sciatica a week after lifting a hose.* This case reveals how easily poor lifting practices can damage the spine, even if the object is not very heavy. In addition to the back pain and sciatica, the patient experienced numbness in his left leg and a limp. The patient rated his pain as an 8 on a 10-point scale. After a battery of tests, the patient was given trigger point therapy, traction, and a program of adjustments to relieve the pain and increase the strength of muscles and spinal structures. After a month of treatment at three times a week, the pain and numbness had improved dramatically. After one month of treatment, the patient reported a 50% improvement of strength, and a 100% after two months. The patient also did exercises at home.

2) *A 39 year-old accountant suffering from headaches, neck pain, facial numbness, and dizziness.* She experienced five headaches every week that were described "like a vice" and were made worse by stress. She took 2 to 4 aspirin a day, but wasn't sure if it made a difference. About two months before seeing a chiropractor, she'd had an episode where her vision blurred, she became shaky, and felt feint. The patient said that it happened during a period of extremely high stress from her job and personal life. After the

incident, she visited a general practitioner and neurologist. As the above symptoms continued, she visited a chiropractor. A diagnosis revealed trigger points and a very prominent misalignment in the cervical vertebrae. The patient had moderate hyperlordosis. After treatments proceeded, intensively for five weeks, the patient reported a 90% improvement of the headaches, a 70% recovery from facial numbness, and a complete recovery from neck pain.

3) *A computer software designer who suffered from a ringing in the ears for 20 years.* He also reported a grinding sound in his neck, "like sandpaper." He experienced neck pain and tension in the jaw muscle. These symptoms were interfering with his work. Upon visiting a upper cervical chiropractor, X-rays revealed a misalignment of his skull in relation to the top (atlas) vertebra. After one adjustment, the grinding sound ceased completely, and the neck pain decreased. The ringing in the ears did not cease, but there had been only 2 adjustments at the time of writing. After these treatments, however, the patient was able to distinguish sounds better, and found that he felt better and more productive in his work.

4) *A 38 year-old nurse who suffered a shoulder injury at work.* Her job is physically demanding, requiring constant motion and a great deal of lifting. The patient suffered from shoulder pain, neck pain, headaches and low back pain. There was a great amount of pressure at the base of the skull, causing significant pain. A regular program of adjustments was ordered, including activator and upper cervical adjustments. She felt relief in the upper neck area and in her shoulder. Her headaches lessened, making her demanding job that much easier.

5) *A 12 year-old girl with head tilt and hyperlordosis.* Children are sometimes forgotten when it comes to considering chiropractic care. This story, however, shows that there is no age requirement

for it. This young girl suffered from headaches in addition to the back and neck pain. Her poor posture was the most likely source of these problems. X-rays showed misalignment of the skull with the atlas vertebra. After one month of Chiropractic treatment, the alignment was corrected and her posture returned to a normal.

Global Chiropractic

Having seen level of satisfaction with chiropractic in the U.S., you may wonder about the rest of the world. Has chiropractic spread from the United States since its inception more than a century ago? Yes, it has.

The World Federation of Chiropractic (WFC) is a large alliance of over 60 countries that benefit from chiropractic. This assembly meets periodically to manage their affairs. Their goals include:

- Acting with national international organizations to provide information and other assistance in the fields of chiropractic and world health.
- Promoting uniform high standards of chiropractic education, research and practice.
- Providing advice on appropriate legislation for chiropractic in member countries.

This organization is an important part of establishing universal standards of education, research, and practice. In education, for example, the Federation has established norms that follow a North American model: entrance requirements to colleges around the world vary with each country, but there is a minimum of two years' university credits qualifying subjects in North America. Although chiropractic colleges once existed only in the United States, there are now colleges in Australia, Brazil, Canada, Denmark, England, France, Japan, Mexico, and others. There are now chiropractic practices in every region of the globe.

The numbers of chiropractors vary. In England, there were 900 practicing chiropractors in 1994. Japan had around 9000 chiropractors in 1997. The United States currently has between 50,000 and 79,000 chiropractors. The law now recognizes chiropractic in all the member countries of the WFC. In general, private health insurance companies provide coverage for chiropractic wherever it has become established. In certain countries, chiropractic enjoys extensive coverage under government health plans: Canada, Denmark, Norway, Sweden, Switzerland, the UK and the United States. All governmental research projects that studied chiropractic have recommended funding for chiropractic services.

Worldwide, then, there is a growing recognition of chiropractic's benefits. There is a move, too, toward a better symbiosis between traditional medicine and chiropractic. In Britain, for example, there is much less friction between the two forms of health care.

Summary and Conclusion

Throughout this text, we have endeavored to make a balanced representation of the methods of adjustment. Since no book can cover every issue, we hope that any unanswered questions you still have will lead you to investigate further. With this presentation, we hope to have given you at least a foothold on this exciting area of health care.

To summarize, there is mounting evidence to support the effectiveness of chiropractic for healing neck pain, back pain, whiplash, and headaches by providing a method of balancing the spine. Chiropractic's philosophy centers on how the musculo-skeletal system of the spine relates to health. Because the spinal cord is the coordinator of the nervous system, it plays a crucial role in regulating bodily systems. If there is a dysfunction in the spine, then, it can have drastic consequences for the body. For instance, the body's built-in mechanism to heal itself can become impaired. Pain is the signal that a problem exists. Often, that problem can be traced to the spine. The chiropractic theory, therefore, holds that by correcting problems within the spine, not only can pain be eliminated, but the *original cause* of the pain as well. Chiropractic also holds the conviction of preventing the degeneration of the spine.

Chiropractic reflects a profoundly compelling notion for many people. Patients around the world have seen how this drugless, non-invasive practice can use the body's natural healing mechanisms to heal. In the end, back pain is not about pain at all, but rather the freedom from it. In the following years, as we learn more about the way the complex systems of the body work, we take steps closer and closer to finding novel, lasting, and humane solution to neck and back pain.

978-0-595-00623-6
0-595-00623-X

www.ingramcontent.com/pod-product-compliance
Lightning Source LLC
Chambersburg PA
CBHW020306290526
45784CB00003B/1383